BODY BREAKDOWNS

BODY BREAKDOWNS

Tales of Illness & Recovery

Edited by Janis Harper

Anvil Press | Vancouver | 2007

Anvil Press Publishers Inc.
P.O. Box 3008, Main Post Office
Vancouver, B.C. V6B 3X5 canada
www.anvilpress.com

LIBRARY AND ARCHIVES CANADA CATALOGUING IN PUBLICATION

  Body breakdowns : tales of illness & recovery / edited by Janis Harper.

ISBN 978-1-895636-86-4

  1. Diseases—Canada. 2. Sick—Canada. 3. Medical care—Canada. 4. Narrative medicine—Canada. 5. Patients' writings. I. Harper, Janis, 1960- II. Title: Tales of illness and recovery.

R726.5.B63 2007   362.10971   C2007-906041-2

Printed and bound in Canada
Interior design: HeimatHouse

Represented in Canada by the Literary Press Group
Distributed by the University of Toronto Press

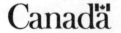 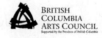 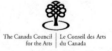

The publisher gratefully acknowledges the financial assistance of the Canada Council for the Arts, the Book Publishing Industry Development Program (BPIDP), and the Province of British Columbia through the B.C. Arts Council and the Book Publishing Tax Credit.

CONTENTS

Preface

My body began breaking down a few years ago, not long after I entered my forties, and I found myself in the hospital, having to surrender my body to strangers. I've always been proudly independent, and there I was, suddenly vulnerable, at the mercy of surgeons and nurses and confronting my mortality. I never admitted that I was scared. But I was. And I might have felt less afraid and isolated if I'd known that other people had similar experiences, shared some of the same kinds of fears. I needed to hear their stories. I needed a book like this one.

Here are very personal, very true stories written by people who have experienced various kinds of body breakdowns; they are about people discovering they're vulnerable as they age and the different ways they come to terms with that. Here are stories about interactions with the medical world, about living with pain both chronic and temporary, and about what it means to be sick or healthy or facing death. They are also about how people who have physically suffered learn to find words for, and thus form, the new worlds they find themselves in.

My hospital visit culminated in the removal of my entire large colon; then, a few years later, my gall bladder had to go. My digestive system was being dismantled, organ by organ. But I couldn't talk about it—there were no words for it; it was too much, too on the brink of life and death. I had ceased to be myself. And if I wasn't myself, how could I talk to other people?

Our bodies are our first means of expression, and they shape how we interact with the world—how we see the world, and how it sees us. When we're young, we're invincible: The world is ours, we can do anything. As we age, our bodies begin to tell us that we have limitations. Sometimes the world shrinks to just the body, as it demands attention from us. We learn, sometimes suddenly and often painfully, that without the body, there's no world. The body breakdown is thus a breaking down of order in the world, of familiar structures of perception. When the body fails, everything falls apart.

Those of us who have experienced body breakdowns eventually learn how to build our own narratives, ways to explain what happened to us. We tell our stories and retell them because we need to: The telling helps us recover from our illness by ascribing order and coherence—that is, "reality"—to an otherwise unreal experience. It helps us recover the world.

We also tell our stories because we find out that others really do want to hear them: This is what happened to me; what happened to you? We want to know, not only because we might get some useful information, not just for pragmatic reasons, but because we can relate—that's all. We all have one. The body is the ultimate common denominator.

Our bodies falling apart bring us together. Brad Zembic, whose story about hernia surgery begins this anthology, discovers "the breakdown of body is what bonds me to living. I'm no longer a master, just part of everything." And in Susan Olding's story about hypertension she observes that if death is the "Great Leveller," sickness is also "a democracy. We will all participate in it one day." Indeed.

For some of us, middle age is our passport to a foreign world populated by practitioners who speak a strange language, yet whose job it is to know our bodies more intimately than we do. And as J. Cates reminds us in his advice to the boomers ("who are beginning to crash upon the medical profession like waves on rocks"), "Medical people are working stiffs like any other and will sometimes screw up." So Alan Girling writes about the problems of medical diagnosis, and both Kim Clark and Ruth Murdoch negotiate the difficult terrain between their experience and what their doctors tell them.

In the public sphere, where we glorify health and wellness, being sick is considered bad, wrong, a symptom of personal failure. After all, maybe it's really *our* fault our bodies fail us: Something's out of whack; our energy is unbalanced; we're not in harmony with the universe. Or our immune system isn't working as it should because years of suppressed emotion have weakened it. Somehow, we've lost control of ourselves. Illness is therefore something we might be ashamed of, or, in any case, want to keep private. When Melody Hessing submitted her story about fracturing her hip, she wrote in her cover letter, "I have long thought that deconstructions of the everyday corporal, from hemorrhoids to heart surgery to hip replacements, deserve more public attention. The Olympic Games are staged for so-called 'excellence'; funerals attend death; but the awkward, humbling, and sometimes terrifying disintegration of flesh and bone remain much too private."

This book attempts to make the private public, to take the awkward, humbling, and sometimes terrifying out of the claustrophobic hospital ward, the hushed doctor's office, the darkened bedroom, and into the sunlight and fresh air. Always reflective, sometimes funny, occasionally disturbing—and whether about a sprained knee, a wrong diagnosis, or multiple sclerosis—these stories remind us that everything can change in a moment. And that we're all in these aging bodies together.

—*Janis Harper, Vancouver, B.C.*

49

Brad Zembic

Forty-nine. Leaving my fifth decade of existence. In thirty years I may be like my father—riddled with diagnoses and preparing to greet God Almighty. Forty-nine. Only a few weeks left, but my body's racing ahead. I'm just back from having some bloody hospital test, plugged into a machine I can't remember the name of. Too many syllables. I'm not like my parents or older friends who rattle them off like they all have medical degrees. I'm still a newbie at forty-nine, a child learning to speak the language of aging.

"It's as bad as having a baby, eh?" a guy sitting next to me says on my second-ever visit to a hospital. The first was at my birth. That's right—forty-nine years ago. This time it's to have a kidney stone removed. Until I had one of my own, I thought "ultrasound" referred to some type of hi-fi technology, like Dolby.

"Fifty percent of people who get stones come back with more, ya know," he adds. Not me, I think, grinning. This is a one-off thing. After today, it's back to normal. A month later, though, a prodding doctor asks me how long I've had my inguinal hernia. A scene from a 1970's sitcom flicks through my brain: a group of cock-wagging men sitting in an office, snickering about why a co-worker had to take some time off. I grew up knowing instinctively that a hernia had to do with *down there*, that it was something to be embarrassed

about. It was a different doctor who told me I actually had two—
one ready to pop, the other still in gestation. Twins, he joked.
Joined at the hip.

When I turned forty, older friends said it was a magical age
when everything starts to make sense; it's when life really begins,
they promised. Now that I'm about to add another full decade to
my count, they're saying this *new* number is when life starts.
Could be it's all in the mind. Nothing to do with consolidating
years of lessons in living. The body goes; the brain tags along. Or
perhaps it's the other way around. Maybe that's why a lot of older
people appear so placid, so self-accepting. They simply don't have
the neural connections to make a fuss about things. But I'm not
there, yet. I'm only forty-nine. I'm still twenty years younger than
my dear friend Jane was when we first met. She's gone now, lived
until the dawn of the new millennium. I didn't understand then
the tribulations of her aged physicality: Her failing eyesight, her
edema, and eroding body were part of a natural progression I
never paid attention to.

But now here I lie. On a cloud-white bed with wheels. I'm ready to
go under the knife as they say. I'm going to be given an anaesthetic.
Something to make me unaware of the sharp-edged implement that
will slice an entrance to my inner world. I'm beginning to feel mortal for a change. Near me there's an old man—over forty-nine, at any
rate—who looks remarkably like Jane. His hair is wiry and grey, his
eyes the creamy blue of the elderly. We talk for a moment, brothers
in experience, but his voice echoes none of her refined English accent
or self-assuredness. A nurse appears from behind a set of curtains.
She hovers over me, checking my blood pressure, and I gaze up at
her like a baby in a crib. It's time.

It's a short journey to the operating room where resplendent haloes of light hang from the ceiling. Tubes are attached; an oxygen mask slips over my face. I could be giving birth I muse. A caesarian. Then, as if time skipped forward, I'm surrounded by gurneys of blue-smocked patients in various stages of recovery. The joy of modern medicine—unlike giving birth, you get to sleep through the whole damn thing. For the next week, though, I move painfully around my downtown apartment, thinking any step will reopen my wound, that my entrails will jack-in-the-box onto the Turkish carpet.

At the high school where I teach, one of my students asks me why I've been away. In university I was trained to seize the teachable moments. I sketch a child-like picture on the blackboard, complete with groin, stomach, and protruding intestine. I'm careful to omit the sexual organ—one doesn't want to be caught drawing penises on blackboards at my age. I think my explanation of how a hernia develops is very clear, but later a colleague approaches me, giggling. "Your student tells me you were in the hospital because you couldn't keep it up." I guess he saw the same sitcom.

Forty-nine is a significant number—a number of transition. In Tibetan Buddhism, it's the number of days someone spends in *bardo*, the state between incarnations. For Kabbalists, passing through the forty-ninth Gate of Understanding opens one to true self-knowledge. I'm in the middle. Between selves. In a few weeks, I'll be a new person. My world will be different. My steps, I imagine, will be lighter, filled with grace—Mother Mary come to me— when I leave my fifth decade of being. The spirit grows as the body crumbles.

At night, I inspect my scar. It appears straight-lipped and foreboding. Eventually the baldness around it will sprout a fresh beard of pubic hair. I rub my finger over my left groin. It's imperceptible, but I know it's there, growing like a fetus—my right hernia reincarnated. I'm being patched like a worn inner tube. Too many bumpy kilometres on the road of life. Spinning through years of personal stress: sibling rivalries and the confused sexual identity of my youth; then an adulthood filled with feelings of inadequacy, romantic disillusionment, the endless search for comfort. And now, RRSP contributions.

What's left but body breakdown? The invisible inside. Around me people appear healthy and fit. They run, they rollerblade, they carry heavy groceries from supermarkets. I watch them as the dotted white man lights my way to the other side of Pacific Boulevard. I ease myself onto the street, hoping to cross before the flaming red hand pulsates its warning. But my groin throbs with pain, and I walk not as a forty-nine-year-old but as someone much older. I'm only halfway to the opposite curb when a black BMW pulls up to me. Its engine is growling and the driver's face curiously reminds me of a bulldog's. "Fucking asshole!" he barks as he tries to regain the six seconds of life he lost waiting for me.

There *is* a gate. I can feel it in my body. My doctor, who has seen me more in the past year than he has in the last twenty, tells me I need to have—get this—an esophagogastroduodenoscopy. They stick a bloody tube down your throat with a camera attached. In my case it's to find out why I'm on a steady diet of antacids. This time I go to the hospital reception like I'm checking into a familiar hotel. I'm given a gown and slippers and told I'm third in line. People are actually lining up for this thing. In the OR, I'm given an anaesthetic. A plastic funnel is strapped to my mouth. The next thing I know, a nurse is shepherding me out the front door. "We had to take a biopsy, but everything else is okay." Wham bam, good luck, man. Now I'm left wondering if my next gate will be made of pearl.

Whatever it is, I know it will open to a different place. I'll be reborn no matter what. Either I'll be in the downward spiral or the upward one—maybe both simultaneously. It puts a burning in my belly, though. A feeling that spreads like the warmth of good wine. There's a connection with life that, I believe, only comes with experiencing its fragility. I can already see through it. The next gate is a gate of consciousness. Of relationship. It's where I embrace the notion that separateness is fiction. The breakdown of body is what bonds me to living. I'm no longer a master, just part of everything. I look at the unborn hernia in my left groin, then at the scar from my surgery. I tug the ends of the fine pink line upward, coaxing a smile.

Saving Time

Emma Kivisild

C all me middle-aged. The label fits. In the middle of my aging. Grey hair, bad memory, need rest. Call me diseased. That too. Multiple sclerosis eating my myelin sheaths. Call me lame—I use a cane, my left leg doesn't work right. But call me beautiful as I stand looking down the concrete steps.

I hear the pneumatic tools in the garage across the road. I hear the cars and their brakes as they approach the intersection. The crossing signal for the blind is chirping.

The steps reach from the terraced garden to the sidewalk, and the terrace makes a concrete ledge on either side. There are nine steps. There is no rail, but if I make it down four steps, the ledge will be at the right height for me to reach under the bush and lean on it. If I can reach that ledge, the steps will be easy.

Or. I can turn back now and go the back way. No steps there.

It is longer and slower the back way. No one who could walk right would go the back way. No one goes the back way but me. Today I am saving time.

Call me reckless. Call me stupid. Call me brave as I stand here.

I take the first step down: left, right, together, pause, and rest on cane. Only three steps now.

Call me terrified for the split second when my foot catches and I lurch. Do I lurch? I feel a lurch. There can't be a lurch because if there were, I would be tumbling, banging, and scraping on the steps. I would be at the foot trying not to cry. This lurch is a warning terror telling me to go back, but I don't.

Why would someone who fell on her face on the flat, tiled kitchen floor only last night be trying these steps? There is no need.

You can call me whatever you want. The lurch is over. Only three steps. I'm dreaming the impossible dream, here. Don't get in my way.

I am making good time.

Remember? Remember when time was something I made? Not something that stretched before me, waiting to be filled, not always a sensible, measured, sluggish pace. Time was varied. I could do close, explosive urgency; brisk distance; long, silky dawdling. I varied it myself. I made it good if I wanted to.

If only time were elastic again. I wish for rushing, hurrying, running late, cutting it close. Instead time has stretched itself fixed, an old waistband that has to be tightened with a safety pin.

I am still learning to choose *slow* by default, so humour me when I pretend I have the need for other options. Let me do this front steps thing.

Middle age and MS are hard to tell apart, sometimes. Which one is responsible for my dulling memory, my worsening eyesight? I am hardly the only middle-aged woman I know with a cane. Does it matter why I have one? Maybe not. I'm too old to be a prodigy, too old to be up-and-coming, too old to make an entrance and set tongues wagging. Too bad at walking to discover a new city on my own. Too old to start a career.

Maybe not too old. People go to law school in their forties. It's the MS that means I can't work full-time. Can't see the small print. Can't take on an exciting heavy workload. Need to sleep every afternoon. It is true that I have been woefully inept at seizing opportunity in my life, but I have enjoyed living the potential in my mind. I have thrilled to the fantasy of meeting famous people I admire. I have dreamt of climbing hills and towers. I have wondered at pictures of beautiful, inaccessible beaches. But now, instead of an unfurling stream of images, I get *can't can't can't.*

To fight the *can'ts*, I've embraced slackerhood, replaced *can't* with *won't*. I would rather be charming and indolent than old and disabled. I do this even though I know that no one is fooled.

The worst is when someone asks, "What do you do?"

I'm middle-aged, I have a disability, I take the front stairs sometimes, I think.

"You're living with multiple sclerosis," a friend tells me. "That's your job."

Nothing was snatched from me. I am alive right now.

Left, right, together, pause. And again and again. I lean perilously to the bushy ledge and plant my hand in the dirt. I fairly skip down the last steps. If you can call it skipping. I do it, anyway. Call me spectacular as I stand still for a moment before I let go and weave down the sidewalk to the intersection.

Numbness Ain't What It Used to Be

Grant Buday

What irritates me about carpal tunnel syndrome is not the numbness in my hands. I could cope with that. I could even get to like it. To me, numbness means comfort, the jagged edges smoothed away until all is as soft and welcoming as a feather bed. This is numbness as it should be, a form of escape. And escape, contrary to our cultural ethos, is good.

"Numb" is supposed to mean "no pain." Codeine makes you numb; the dentist gives you novocaine to numb your teeth, to escape the pain of reality. Or is it the reality of pain? My carpal tunnel isn't like that; mine hurts like a toothache in my elbow, and this just isn't right. My numbness burns, prickles, and throbs. My fingers are furred with a numbness that pinches. Life without escape is, well, work. That wise, fast-driving Frenchman, Albert Camus, said that Sisyphus' only escape from pushing that boulder up the hill for all eternity was to learn, somehow, to enjoy pushing it up that hill. No doubt masochism is an option for some of us.

I'm still working on escape. But carpal tunnel syndrome compromises both work and escape. According to my research, carpal tunnel syndrome occurs when the median nerve, which runs from the forearm into the hand, becomes pressed or squeezed at the wrist.

The median nerve controls sensations to the palm side of the thumb and fingers, as well as impulses to some small muscles in the hand that allow the fingers and thumb to move. The carpal tunnel is a narrow passageway of ligament and bones at the base of the hand. Thickening from irritated tendons narrows the tunnel and causes the median nerve to be compressed.

In chronic and/or untreated cases, the muscles at the base of the thumb may waste away. Some people are unable to tell between hot and cold by touch.

Now, I don't want to hear—or read with my bifocals—this sort of thing. Carpal tunnel, blood pressure, cholesterol, and arthritis are starting to rival money, sex, travel, and dreams of glory as dominant themes of conversation with my contemporaries. All too soon I'll be like seniors I know, engrossed by the progress of their own decay and that of their friends—for someone they know is inevitably going through "a procedure," having tests, dealing with kidneys, lungs, Alzheimer's, feet, or cancer. The list goes on, and so do they. What they need is a holiday, an escape—from themselves—the numbing sunshine of a long bland cruise from nowhere to nowhere.

The inescapable fact of mortality makes some people mature. They take on a warm glow like a sunset and emanate a soft yet penetrating radiance born of wisdom. Not me. I'm bitter. I'd flagellate my traitorous body but for the fact that it would only make it break down even faster. I'm hoping that the masses of wealthy baby boomers are frantically pumping piles of dough into geriatrics research so that by the time I'm a senior, there will be a range of tasty treatments awaiting people with carpal tunnel syndrome—such as new and improved hormone therapies, delightful diets involving pastries, spa weekends featuring baths in Nilotic mud, and dolphin-oil massages performed by young ladies. Who knows, it may turn out that at fifty-one I've barely reached middle age!

While I may not be wise and radiant, I have discovered one very effective and unfairly maligned life skill: blaming others. My carpal tunnel syndrome is directly attributable to Captain Bligh, who lives up the road. He is a fisherman who, in the off season, instead of taking it easy, instead of dabbling in water colours, believes he must do carpentry—and for some strange reason, he thinks I should do carpentry too. Recently he needed help tearing out a kitchen for some unsuspecting elderly couple. I should have been true to my first and wisest urge, which was to avoid, but like so many good men, I was led astray by the lure of cash. Plus, I envisioned joyously smashing old kitchen cabinets with a crowbar, childishly glorying in destruction like the ape with the bone at the start of *2001: A Space Odyssey*—and being paid for it. Instead I got stuck wheelbarrowing gyproc, wood, a dishwasher, and all too many large cabinets up a steep driveway. The next day I tore up the floor, which involved extensive work with a six-foot steel bar. And then lugging it all up that ever-steeper, ever-longer driveway in that wheelbarrow. Sustained gripping. With weight. A bad combination.

The back, legs, and shoulders were fine. But the hands . . .

As is often the case with chronic pain, my carpal tunnel has become a creature in its own right, and in my case, it is nasty, vindictive, resentful, and vicious, especially when aggravated. (I have begun to suspect that chronic pain, like a pet, begins to resemble its owner.) When the carpal tunnel beast hibernates, I can make it through the night waking only a couple of times. But when it rages, as it did after working with Captain Bligh, I was up no less than seven times. Not merely awake, but out of bed and pacing, because only being upright for at least ten minutes can gradually soothe the surly animal. Furthermore, there is only one position in which I am permitted to doze off: on my left side, right arm carefully arranged, like a prosthesis.

Please understand that for me, an escapist, a devotee of avoidance, sleep is akin to numbness. And I love them both. Sleeping has long been one of my favourite activities; there was a time in my life when it seemed like the only reward for slogging through yet another futile day. Sleep meant not merely a brief escape, but oblivion, settling like an exhausted flatfish into the sweet, soft silt at the bottom of my unconscious. Not surprisingly, my taste in drugs has always leaned toward opiates. To be deprived of something as fundamental as sleep, something I so dearly love, is doubly anguishing. No numbness for you, my lad, no escape: You stay here, awake, in pain, condemned to consciousness, condemned to your own company. No escape. This is my definition of hell.

I can state with confidence that the adage about pain making man think and thinking making man wise is false. Pain blots out thought, dominating the mind with its siren blare.

Treatment? Of course there is a treatment. It's called surgery. And by all accounts, it does not work. Or it does for six months and then everything is back, only worse. Still, you've had a nice little hospital stay—ah, the décor, the yawning nurses, the non-union cleaning staff, the powdered potatoes, tinned meat, and scalding tea—you've had a lot of ineffective and constipating pain killers, plus you have an anecdote to inflict on people until, that is, they turn their hearing aids off.

Not that having carpal tunnel is all bad. It saved me from a nervous breakdown at the age of nineteen. At the time, I had a job standing at the end of a ripsaw, stacking two-by-tens. There seemed to be a great demand for two-by-tens in those days.

Perhaps there still is, I don't know, for having been permanently traumatized, I avoid two-by-tens the way some people avoid pitbulls. A strange little man stood at the other end of the saw, shoving wood through, while I stacked the pieces that emerged from the shrieking steel blades. He was a stout chap with a hardhat and a carpenter's pencil in the breast pocket of his overalls—a pencil that he used to clean his ears and perhaps add the occasional semi-literate verse to a crudely illustrated obscene epic on the toilet wall. Either way, there I was in the satanic mill: the machines racketing, the ripsaw shrieking, the wood rushing relentlessly at me. And there was no way out. Or not one with any dignity, and in those days I still clung to quaint notions of dignity and pride. My life was over, I would stack two-by-tens forever, the best I could ever achieve would be to one day take the place of the strange little man on the other end of the saw, in my own overalls, cleaning my ears with my own carpenter's pencil, pushing wood in rather than pulling wood out.

By great good fortune, at this very same time, my hands were busy going numb. I promptly parlayed it into a doctor's appointment; the wise physician sent me to the specialist, who hooked me up to electrodes. Thank God for electrodes. Prognosis: Quit that job. The man likely still remembers the nineteen-year-old who fell to the floor and hugged his knees. For this I will always be grateful to my carpal tunnel.

But, some thirty years later, I must accept the fact that it doesn't take two-by-tens to make my hands numb. Holding a pen or chopsticks or a hammer will do it. My hands become foreign objects, and my fingers turn into strangely burning digits that refuse to do what they're told. Worse, there is no more escaping this condition than one can escape death. Just as the greying hair indicates that I've used up my quotient of pigment cells, I must accept the reality that my body is wearing out, and that not even good old numbness, not even the absence of sensation, can be relied upon to let you slip out the side door and avoid the whole bad business.

The Other Country

Susan Olding

D r. Corbeau made me sick. She flew into the examining room, her dark hair shimmering, her shrewd eyes scanning the scratch marks on my chart, her small hands with their sharp nails riffling through the pages. The mere sight of her made me nervous, but since she was one of the few doctors accepting new patients in the city I'd recently moved to, I couldn't afford to be picky. My jaw tightened at the pitch of her voice, so insistent, so acerbic, so anxious. Ten days ago she had announced that my blood pressure was too high and she was taking me off the Pill.

Timidly, I said, "My sex life."

"You should get an IUD," she said.

My jaw dropped. She shrugged and thrust some pamphlets in my hand.

Now I was here for follow-up. From my perch, high on the table, I watched her seize the blue rubber pump. *Breathe*, I told myself. *Deep breaths.* She fastened the cuff round my arm, then tightened it. Her narrow wrist was bronzed from a weekend of tennis. *You should wear sunscreen*, I thought. The cold mouth of the stethoscope jolted me. The needle surged.

Her eyes narrowed. "You did stop taking those pills?"

"Of course." My pulse was knocking.

Shaking her head, she pumped again, then dropped the rubber bulb as if it had burned her.

"That's it. Get down. Get out of here. Get to the hospital." Beneath its tan, her face was pale. She scribbled her readings on a sheet of blue paper.

"Do you understand? Get to the hospital *now*. You're going to stroke on me."

Stroke. The word slammed like an iron bar or a steel door between us, blocking thought, blocking all possibility of communication. Stroke. *People die of that.* Stroke. *But I'm not old!* Stroke. *And I'm not ill!*

I was thirty-two, slim, a non-smoker, a moderate drinker, with no history of stroke or heart disease in the immediate family, with no risk factors at all, other than a decade's worth of carefully monitored oral contraceptive use. Apart from visits to the doctor, I'd never felt better.

Get to the hospital. What can Dr. Corbeau have been thinking? How did she expect me to get there? Was I supposed to drive? I hadn't brought a car. What can *I* have been thinking? Why didn't I call a taxi? But I didn't. Instead, clutching the note she'd given me in sweaty fingers, with a dazed stupidity that still astonishes me, I walked the two miles to the local emergency room.

A pair of young residents took charge of me. While one drew blood and delivered it to the lab to be screened for possible secondary causes, the other cuffed me again, and asked some questions. "Any unusual headaches? Blurry vision? Dizziness?"

No. No. And no. "Sometimes after my run, if it's really hot outside, I feel a little woozy."

"You *run*?" He frowned. "I don't understand these readings. Right now . . . the pressure's a bit higher than normal . . . but nothing like the figure your doctor quoted. I'm going to leave you for half an hour and see what happens." When he returned, he shrugged at me. "It's gone down. Borderline, I'd say. Go back to

Dr. Corbeau in a couple of days. She may suggest medication."

Ordinarily we think of illness and disease as identical and use the words interchangeably, but as medical historian Jacalyn Duffin reminds us, philosophers find it helpful to distinguish between the concepts. For them, "illness" refers to an individual's experience of suffering; "disease" refers to the *theory* used to explain the illness, to define its presumed causes, and to describe the paths it will take.

Not ill, I had said to myself in Dr. Corbeau's examining room. Nor was I, if "illness" equals suffering. Still, I left the hospital stamped with a new label and a new identity. *Hypertensive*. Hypertension is a disease, a chronic and potentially threatening condition. In pamphlets issued by the Heart and Stroke Foundation, it is called a "silent killer." I imagine it as a bird of prey, a raptor. Since that June afternoon, my blood pressure has fluctuated, mostly within the normal range, but even at its lowest, it is higher than average, and visits to the doctor send it soaring. "White Coat Syndrome," this is called. Researchers disagree about its significance, but surely such sensitivity suggests pathology of some description. Should I salt my food less, refuse that extra glass of wine? Should I be taking medication? The questions hover, unspoken, but never beyond awareness. More accurately than many of us, I can predict my ultimate end. The insult to the brain, the sudden affront to the heart.

Before modern technology, a "disease" such as hypertension, unaccompanied by "illness," was literally unthinkable. But suffering without explanation, "illness" without "disease," has long been with us. About a year ago, I received an overdue letter from a friend in another part of the country. She apologized for being such a poor correspondent; she'd had some health problems; she hoped I'd understand. The trouble began with a strange ache in her breast while she was nursing her second daughter. At first she feared cancer, but fortunately, a series of tests had ruled out that diagnosis. Meanwhile, the pain spread, first to her arms, and then to her legs. Her doctors began to investigate for multiple sclerosis or another disease of the central nervous system. But that trail also ended in a blank wall.

Some days, my friend can't type; she is a lawyer, so she finds this inconvenient. Some days she cannot tie her daughters' shoes; she is the mother of two toddlers, and so the ache in her heart competes with the ache in her fingers. Her pain is real, and really debilitating, but she does not *look* unwell, and she is growing tired of the doubt she reads in people's eyes. Now her doctors are talking about a virus, or fibromyalgia, or depression. Especially depression. "They think it's all in my head," she says. "Yes, I'm depressed. *Of course* I'm depressed. They'd be depressed, too, if they hurt all the time and nobody believed them!"

Chronic conditions threaten the well, and undiagnosed chronic conditions, like my friend's, threaten the well most profoundly. Chronic conditions defeat sympathy: *Get over it, already!* Chronic conditions invite blame: *It's just her personality.* Chronic conditions challenge the reigning, and therefore comfortable, conception of disease as ontological—something separate from us, coming from outside, and capable of defeat. Chronic conditions are not so much something we "have" as something we "are."

Or something we become. My friend's undiagnosed disease, her inexplicable illness, is a constantly hovering presence. She has worse days and better days, but even at her best, she is never as she once was. Still, that doesn't imply she is *less*. The neurologist Oliver Sacks writes about his patients' "creative adaptations" to their problems—the ways they "reach out to life—not only despite their conditions, but often because of them, and even with their aid."

We are all familiar with the more mundane examples: the myopic child, no good at sports, who becomes an avid reader; the uncle whose heart condition induces him to walk, and whose walks awaken the amateur ornithologist in him. Suffering may not ennoble, but inevitably it changes our perspective.

An aunt of mine, following a brave and ultimately successful battle with breast cancer, remarked to me that although her family's love and support had been important to her throughout her ordeal, she had come to see her struggle as a journey that must be undergone alone. At most she might share parts of it with other survivors. No one who had not "been there" could offer much in the way of aid; no one who had not "been there" could fully understand.

Illness *is* another country. If the land of health can be conceived of as an aristocracy, where the best genes win, or as a meritocracy, where you are what you eat, and your condition reflects your habits, then illness is an oligarchy, in which the many (our witty phrases, our skill at knitting, our perfect pitch, the pressure of our tread on the stair) are ruled by the few (the germs that have invaded us, our inherited vulnerabilities). At its worst it becomes a tyranny. Yet death, they say, is the Great Leveller, and so sickness is also, and always, a democracy. We will all participate in it one day. Meanwhile, our doctors in their bright white coats guard the borders, their machines anxiously shrieking the alarm whenever one of us slips past.

Dropping the blood pressure gauge in her office that day, Dr. Corbeau had stared at me as if I might be dangerous. Hypertension is not infectious, of course—and if it were, I'm convinced that the contagion must have spread in the opposite direction. But Dr. Corbeau wasn't taking chances. *How dare you*, her expression said— as if I had demanded dual citizenship of unfriendly neighbouring states, states requiring sole and mutually exclusive allegiance.

Behind her indignation I read fear. "You're going to stroke on *me*." Leaving her responsible. No wonder she was anxious. But there was more. "*You're* going to stroke on me." I—a woman of comparable age, class, appearance, education—not old, nor poor, nor fat, nor ignorant—was going to stroke on her. The army of disease was encroaching, too close for safety or for comfort.

She needn't have worried. The diseased don't think of the well that way. They don't want to take them over, or take them along. They don't want to go themselves. Walking from her office to the hospital, wondering if that walk would be my last, wondering if I'd have a chance to say goodbye to the people I love, it was the light I noticed most. Hard and glinting on the main street, filtered and green on the side roads leading to the lake. The breeze, pungent with the smell of someone's newly painted shutters, rustled the leaves of the maple trees and bent the blades of grass. Swallows swooped and chittered in Edwardian gingerbread. Some children sailed past on bicycles, calling out to one another. My pulse—surely too fast, too loud?—set up an answering cry.

A month ago, I fell sick with the flu. I lay for days in my bed, memorizing the shape of clouds outside the window, memorizing the pattern of stitching on the quilt. I could not work. I could not think. I could not eat. My sense of time collapsed: The hours dragged, interminable, or else they galloped and the day disappeared before I knew it had begun.

One morning, I woke at dawn to the clamour of crows. Raucous, insistent, clanging, their alarm went on and on. Our yard is deep and thickly treed; in addition to birds, it is home to mice and skunks and racoons, but to these the crows are ordinarily indifferent. Were I healthy, I would have been actively curious about the cause of their distress; ill, I was no more than dully aware. My ears, already thrumming from infection, hardly registered the insult. I tried to read, I swallowed aspirin, I dozed.

In the afternoon, my neighbour called. "I know you're sick, but I thought you might like to know. There's a Great Horned Owl in your spruce tree."

"So that's what's been bothering the birds."

"Go and take a look at him."

I bundled myself in a sweater and went outside.

The crows had given up; the yard was silent except for the crunch of twigs beneath my feet. I squinted through eyes swollen and crusted with conjunctivitis. The owl perched in magnificent imperturbability midway up the tree. His feathers—golden, brown, and grey—glowed in the weak winter sun. He watched me coolly as I circled the ground beneath him, his body entirely still, his big head swivelling in its socket, his amber eyes unblinking. Such conservation of energy, such concentration of power! In less than a second, he might have left his perch and clamped his talons into me or any other creature moving through the garden. But he did not—not this time. Instead, at fall of dark, he flew, his great wings throwing shadows across the roofs and the parks and the roadways of our city, mapping his mysterious path, back to the country he came from.

Extreme Piles

Bob Wakulich

It is an unfortunate limitation of the human condition that if everyone in the world became totally empathetic, no one would get much accomplished. In such a case, getting out of bed in the morning and casually putting on a pot of coffee in front of people who would like to and can't manage it would be considered a regrettable act of insensitivity.

Luckily, we aren't wired to share pain that way, and consequently, there are times when the witnessing of relative health and vitality can be very depressing. I've been told that migraine sufferers have no trouble understanding this. Exquisite, relentless pain reduces your outlook to a search for relief of the spirit imprisoned by your ailing flesh. Anyone with the slightest bit of credibility could probably convince you that sucking on your family pet's tail might help.

I've found myself experiencing this reaction to the world lately. It's not because of migraines—heck, I'm pretty sure they're nothing compared to this—but from recent hemorrhoid surgery. I'm a veteran when it comes to piles, and when the doctor told me that mine had thrombosed, I knew that was bad and meant something more radical than salves, suppositories, and natural laxatives.

Until I finally went under the knife, I was one of those people you've encountered, the kind who either sit at skewed angles and prop their feet up on chairs all akimbo or who sit rigidly and carry a small pillow under one arm and talk about the fibre content of snack tables and do not laugh at Preparation H jokes.

It's not a condition that people like to discuss, possibly because it tends to put everyone in a lower colonic frame of mind, which isn't conducive to much of anything. Recounting a gruesome episode of mental illness over a cheese tray isn't likely to put too many people off their dinners, but rectal swelling, no matter how delicately related, makes everybody's teeth clench.

You can't blame them. It's hard enough to get hemorrhoid sufferers to talk amongst themselves. Sometimes you'll recognize the symptoms in a stranger across the room, your eyes will meet, you'll nod slightly in recognition, and then you'll receive a cold, measured stare that means, in no uncertain terms, that you shouldn't go there; things are bad enough without exchanging notes.

I managed to dodge the surgery for a while. The previous two specialists—officially, they're proctologists, but I've taken to calling them "bumologists"—told me that a few of the swellings were too close to the end of the line. This was mixed in with talk of mucous membranes, stool softeners, and oat bran, and I was introduced to the concept of small enemas, whatever those are.

Essentially, hemorrhoids are the anal equivalent of varicose veins: Small bundles of free-floating blood vessels form, get jostled, and grow, eventually causing pressure and pain. Sometimes they go away on their own. Sometimes they can be tied with rubber bands and eventually fall off, a relatively simple procedure involving some unusual postures in the doctor's office and a few days of waddling.

If that isn't possible, surgical incisions have to be made: They burrow in, remove the offending veins, and cauterize the area. You can imagine how much fun this is. But by the time this becomes mandatory, you're not really having much fun anyway, getting up three hours early to give yourself enough time to let things calm down before you have to be anywhere.

The procedure itself doesn't take very long. Once you've been prepped and had your legs mounted in straps, it's almost over. Thanks to sedatives and a spinal, I felt great after surgery, better than I'd felt in months, dancing around the nurses' station with an anaesthetic hangover and my pants full of oversized absorbent pads.

Then the drugs wore off. Imagine feeling like you have to go to the bathroom for ten days straight. Imagine trying to pass a ratchet set once a day. Imagine a handheld showerhead becoming your most treasured home appliance.

They give you drugs to take at home, but they're lousy drugs with all kinds of side effects that make you feel squishy and stupid. They also constipate you, so you take mineral oil and eat whatever works in a blender. Standing hurts, sitting hurts, lying down hurts, a ringing telephone hurts, and sneezing is truly an adventure.

It takes about three weeks before you even begin to feel close to normal. Meanwhile, the bumologist is seeing you every four or five days, taking another look, and reminding you that this isn't a part of your body that you can put in a sling. The muscles down there seem to interact with everything. Think about this. Try touching your toes. Try swallowing.

To pass the time, you begin planning what you're going to do when everything settles: no more crossword puzzles, no more gelatin, no more buying bargain toilet paper. What keeps you going is that you look forward to the day when you don't get offended by people who don't have to give a lot of thought to their bowel movements. I'm certain now that this day is coming—though if you'd asked me last week, I may not have been so sure.

Admissions

Adrienne Mercer

It's Kurdish New Year 2003, and I am at a celebration at a community centre in Kitsilano, near my friends Alisa and James' apartment. The organizer, a friend of James, invites us to take part in a simple traditional dance where friends join hands and step sideways in a circle. I am thirty-two and on the waiting list for a knee replacement.

To get to this celebration we walked for fifteen minutes. Later we will need to walk home. To dance tonight will make tomorrow unbearable, and I need to be mobile for my bus and ferry trip home to Vancouver Island. I encourage Alisa and James to go ahead, and they join a festive circle that includes toddlers in pull-ups and elderly folk with canes and gnarled hands. They laugh and chat as they dance, looking over at me and smiling, including me as much as they can. When the party ends, I buy a CD by a Kurdish folk singer named Ahmet Kaya. In the years to follow I will play it often in my apartment, swaying gently as he sings, remembering the dance.

Now it is April 2006, and the hospital clerk on the phone has bad news.

"Adrienne," she says gently, "I've had to cancel your knee surgery. You didn't tell us you were pregnant."

The distance between us seems to lengthen, so that my response, when uttered, falls through the telephone receiver and into a long, deep well.

"I'm not pregnant," I answer, shocked, my voice wavering down the line to her waiting ear. After a lifetime of arthritic pain I am used to complications, but I am not prepared for this. I feel both connected to and disconnected from my body. My left knee—the one soon to be fully replaced with an artificial joint—stiffens. My Self hollows, hovering somewhere above the phone as I stare down at my own scalp.

The clerk apologizes in a quiet voice. "I thought you knew," she says. "They told me you knew."

They? They who? The operation was scheduled for a week today. I have been on a waiting list for two years now. Grinding bone-on-bone pain is part of my daily routine.

I pull my voice up from the well.

"Did the hospital say I was pregnant? I have my period. It started yesterday." I shift sideways in my ergonomic chair and rub my abdomen as if to demonstrate the presence of menstrual cramps. Next, out of habit, I move my hand to rub my sore left knee, repeating the same circular motion I have used since I developed juvenile rheumatoid arthritis at the age of three.

The clerk's voice is brisk now. I have just become a problem, an unwanted booking nightmare.

"You filled out a form two days ago at your pre-admission clinic," she tells me. "One of the questions asks if you're pregnant. You ticked 'yes' and you initialled it. We can't operate if you're pregnant. I've given your time to someone else."

Even through my disbelief, the humour of this situation is not lost on me. Given the average age of women who require knee replacements, this kind of mix-up probably doesn't happen much.

I am thirty-four now, not quite middle-aged in calendar years, but in terms of joint damage, I'm geriatric. My medical chart is thicker than those of most senior citizens, and despite several scopes to clean up the damage in the knee joint, despite daily exercises and glucosamine supplements, there is no cartilage remaining in my left knee. Walking, running, cleaning my house—all of it is torture. Even sleep doesn't come easily—each excruciating toss and turn causes the knee joint to lock and painfully jolt me awake.

I do not tell the clerk that I desperately want to be pregnant, that her mistake has triggered a lonesome numbness. I have not yet had children, largely due to circumstance, but also due to the knee and its struggle to bear even my own weight. Knee replacement surgery is hard on patients, and the artificial joints have a lifespan of only fifteen years, so no doctors wanted to operate before I was forty. Finally, they concurred that carrying a child on the bad knee would be too painful for me, and the best thing to do would be to operate and allow the knee to heal before I began to consider pregnancy.

"There's been a mistake," I say. It takes tremendous effort to sound calm, but I need to fix this, and to do so I must be polite. I explain that the only medical form I initialled at the hospital was a generic green one that an admissions clerk filled in for me, asking me questions and then checking off the appropriate boxes with small neat ticks. "She did give me the form to look over," I recall. "I didn't get far with it because she'd spelled my name wrong, and when I noticed that, she took the form back to change it. Trust me, I'm not pregnant."

She takes a deep breath, her mouth close enough to the receiver that I hear each stage of her inhale. "It's too late," she says, her exhale a rush of words. "I've rebooked someone else into that spot, an elderly woman. She's just thrilled. We'll slot you in again as soon as possible." She pauses, then adds, "I'm sorry about this."

My eyes scan across my desk, across the files I meant to tackle prior to my five weeks of medical leave. A deserving senior citizen now has my surgery date. This news triggers a memory, exposing a raw gash of guilt.

When I was fifteen, I began taking public transit to high school, partly because my new school was too far to walk to and partly because my knee pain had worsened. Even then I'd had arthritis for twelve years; even then my knee was in worse condition than those of my grandparents. My days started with a morning trek to the bus stop at twenty to eight, a stiff-legged walk up the bus steps, and standing-room only in the aisles. Usually I waited for my classmates to disembark so I could scissor-step safely down to the pavement. Settling into my homeroom desk was sweet relief.

My school was next to a seniors' centre, and the bus stop was situated between the two buildings. By three o'clock I was too exhausted for socializing or even standing. I would sit on the school steps and wait for the 155 bus, watching students and seniors vie for position in the lineup. I'd learned early on that there was no point in jostling for a seat. The disapproving stares of seniors if I dared to sit were enough to keep me standing, absorbing the impact of each bump and jolt with a knee joint that had survived steroid injection, physiotherapy, and a barrage of anti-inflammatory drugs. Lurching down the stairs at my stop, I bitterly hoped that the elderly commuters would understand my quiet sacrifice.

"I need that surgery date," I tell the clerk. "I've been to all of your pre-operative courses. I've taken five weeks off work. I've rented a walker and a cane at the Red Cross."

"But this poor other lady, she's so excited."

"That isn't my problem."

She finally agrees to order a pregnancy test, using serum from the blood I gave during my pre-admission lab work. We hang up. As I wait for a callback from the hospital lab, I can't shake my frustration. I silently review the limitations the knee has forced upon me, the ways it has stolen my youth. Everything in me longs for the chance to fully participate in my life.

Much more than a surgery date has been taken from me. My biological clock warns that I should have had children sooner, but my career and my relationship are still young. While I have been seeking maturity and fulfillment in those areas, my fertility has been declining and my knee joint deteriorating with every step. If I can't keep this surgery date, when will the next one be offered?

When the phone rings, the same clerk's voice greets me on the other end of the line. "Adrienne," she says, "this probably doesn't surprise you, but you're not pregnant. The person who completed your form made a mistake." The absurdity of the moment hits me: In waiting by the phone, I have been putting off a trip to the lavatory to change my menstrual pad.

"And my surgery?"

"Same day, same time," she says. "The other lady was really good about it."

Jubilation. I hang up the phone and exhale.

Later, I reach into my shoulder bag to retrieve the joint replacement workbook I got from the hospital physiotherapist. After my surgery, she said, I will need to learn to walk again, to teach my new joint and my old muscles how to work together to support my weight. I will need to learn balance, timing, and pace. This process, I suspect, will be humbling.

I take a deep breath and open the workbook to a diagram. It depicts a smiling elderly woman who, with the aid of a walker, is taking her first, faltering, post-operative steps.

I'm about to be young.

Diagnosis: Square One

Alan Girling

A hard rain in May beats at the window. My wife is away in Japan and my teenage son is at school. Our cat, who we call Smart, paws at my leg while I type. As far as I know, right now, I don't have cancer. But for five days last spring, as far as I knew, I did.

First, a confession: In my later adult life, I've suffered from mild hypochondria. At forty-seven, I'm not in poor health, but you wouldn't know it from the number of times I see the doctor in a year. Any little pain or discomfort and I'm seeking a diagnosis. I want assurance; I want to be told I'm fine. Whatever the doctor declares is how I measure my well-being. Yet, by their nature, medical professionals invariably, perversely, withhold any such comfort or certitude: They play with my head by hedging, never revealing what they suspect the problem might be, delaying all definite statements until weeks have passed, multiple tests performed. Yes, it's their job to be cautious, but I'm impatient. I draw my own conclusions. And that means, invariably, perversely, that I'm not fine. Internet searches matching symptoms with diseases have led me, more than once or twice, to conclude that death is at the door and ready to knock. I tell my wife my fears, but she's smarter than that. Still, the boy in me cries wolf, not as a joke, but because every boy knows there really are wolves out there in the dark, lying in wait. We are but little lambs in a big bad world, after all.

It was just such a vague pain and discomfort that got me to the clinic last spring, one of those set-ups with a stable of physicians so you never know whom you'll meet. This time, I see an older Asian lady. She's soft and plump and asks with a smile how she can help me today. My description of the pain in my abdomen is, like the pain itself, quite vague. It's a pressure, a burning, a soreness, I tell her. It's right here, over here, sometimes down here. She smiles.

After reviewing my ever-thickening file, she examines me, finds a bit of high blood pressure, and orders, along with some blood work, an ultrasound. Why, I ask. Just to eliminate certain possibilities, she says, which I am left to imagine for myself. With a week to wait before the test, I had time to study up on my own. Suffice to say, I all but sentenced myself to less than a year to live as the most likely scenario.

After the ultrasound test, I'd still have at least another week before getting the results. An ultrasound is a painless ordeal, and from past experience, I expected a friendly but coolly professional staff, and no information. First, they directed me to a small dimly lit room with machinery and a monitor set up next to a paper-covered bed. I sat there in my shame-making gown and saw, posted on the wall, the radiologist's code of ethics. It prohibits them from divulging anything about whatever horrors they may discover. I naturally presumed any radiologist to be intimate with her own code; this message was for us. They know we crave information, but all we get is coyness and longer delays. As if they don't know our true fates.

After a few niceties, I'm down on my side, gown open, while

the radiologist applies an icy KY-like goop to my abdomen. She then runs the wand up, down, in swirls, applies pressure here and there, making me hold my breath at intervals while she snaps her images. At one point, she stops. She pushes the wand against my lower rib cage, on my right side. She stares intently at the screen. She squints, and shakes her head. "Breathe in," she says. "Now out." She shifts the wand. Repeat. Again. Once again.

It went on. Clearly she'd found something. Twisting my head, I could easily see the shifting grey and white blobs on the monitor. I felt like an expectant mother searching vainly for the fetal form of her new baby, except I was anticipating something more like the devil's spawn. Apparently, the radiologist assumed I wasn't trained to decipher these images. She was right. I did, however, have some experience reading facial expressions, and I definitely saw the tension in her brow, a hint of panic in her eyes. "Excuse me," she said, and rushed out of the room.

Moments later, she was back with a colleague. No niceties from this guy, he was all business. After examining the screen for a few intense minutes, he took up the wand, scanned the area himself and rang off a series of questions: Are you feeling pain in your right abdomen? Yes, a bit. Have you noticed blood in your urine? No. Have you lost weight recently? No. He put the wand down. The two exchanged a knowing look.

"Okay," he said, "clean yourself up. We'll get a report off to your doctor. She'll set you up with a specialist and likely arrange an immediate CAT scan."

With no other words of explanation, they both walked out.

So. They'd done their jobs. No information provided, as per the code. Real and explicit information that is, spoken, verbalized, reported information—is best handled by one's personal physician. Except I did have information: I had two very concerned experts finding something serious in a particular location inside my body. I had a set of symptoms with which to make inferences. I also had the necessity of further tests, consultations with a specialist. This was too much information, too much for comfort and not enough for certainty. Could I be blamed this time if I refused to wait, if I went straight home, fired up the computer and began my own investigation?

Google sent me first to wrongdiagnosis.com, an incredible resource for paranoiacs. This site and others told me that the combination of symptoms I was suspected of having—abdominal pain, blood in the urine, weight loss—was often linked together with renal cell carcinoma, that is, a cancer of the kidney. That I didn't actually have two of these symptoms was easy to explain according to the website: As with many cancers, people with kidney cancer could have few symptoms, some, or even none. Then I learned that kidney cancer occurs most often in men, men at middle age or later, like forty-six-year-old men.

A few days later, the clinic calls. Surprisingly, I see the same Asian woman. Yes, a growth has been found. It's approximately six by three centimetres, lodged in my right kidney. Is it cancer? Oh, she can't say that, no. She even laughs, a small nervous laugh, but a laugh nevertheless. She's either uncomfortable with the topic, or I'm clearly worrying way too much. But wait a minute. She looks again at the report. Where *is* the growth exactly? The body of the report mentions an oblong mass in the lower part of my right kidney. In the summary at the bottom, however, "right" has mysteriously changed to "left." Which is it? Right or left? I tell her about my ultrasound, that they concentrated on my right side. It must be my right kidney, I say. That's also where I feel the pain, I say. So here I am, me, the patient, telling my doctor what the actual findings are because the experts over at the ultrasound clinic were unable to produce a competent report. Dare I presume surgeons use these reports to decide where to make their incisions and what to remove from a patient's body?

That weekend, steeped in anxiety and more afraid than ever that the healthcare system was letting me down, I ran five kilometres in a fundraising event for ALS (amyotrophic lateral sclerosis). A colleague at the college I teach at had been diagnosed two years previously. Her name was Bridget. I was her first teaching partner. I didn't know it then, but she would have less than a year to live. Bridget was fifty-two. I knew her as one with tremendous spirit, and as I ran through the wooded parkland, a cold April rain drizzling down, it was hard not to take in some of that spirit, feel the touch of kinship. How much longer could I keep this body going? Though my fate had yet to be sealed, I found I needed, like her, to keep pushing it through to its natural conclusion. The cheers and hugs I got from my work fellows waiting at the finish line helped me recognize one small victory in the journey.

Monday, I saw the specialist, a brash and confident young urologist with short curly hair and a pink boyish complexion. His office window presented a view of the North Shore mountains. I could see the sun reflecting off a patch of snow. If my GP was unable to be forthright about my condition, he certainly wasn't. I had a cancer, and he would do everything possible to effect a cure. "It's not unrealistic," he said. First, though, a CAT scan was needed to help make a proposal for treatment. "Let's get it done right away. Any questions?"

I nodded. I had no questions. I was not in the least surprised. But I began to feel dizzy, could feel my heart pounding. The mountains disappeared; the doctor faded, too—not from sight, but from understanding, engagement. I was being quickly drawn inward into a new and darker zone, far from anything familiar. I heard his voice. The imaging department would call with a time. A time? For the CAT scan. Yes, right, the CAT scan. First, though, I had to go home. I had to tell my wife the news.

I could have said, I told you so, but I felt no satisfaction at having my paranoia validated like this. We just lay on the bed in the afternoon light. She touched my arm and said if I were to die, her life would be over. We'd been married almost twenty years. Still, I felt something like awe, that I could be so important to her. I had trouble believing it. My mortality was a fact to me. I didn't see fully how real it could be to her or anyone else.

I wasn't especially angry at my fate, or not yet. Nor did I begin a mental fight against the possibility of dying young. My hypochondria, it seemed, had brought me closer to an acceptance of early death. Instead of crying, why me, I thought, why not me? I wasn't special. Not that I didn't hold out a bit of hope. I wouldn't mind being a cancer survivor. It had a nice ring to it. Still, my ingrained pessimism failed to steel me completely from the blow. For the first time in my adult life, I cried myself to sleep, thinking of her, but also . . .

. . . my son, fifteen years old. I wanted to see him graduate, marry, make a life for himself. How would my passing affect him? Could I guide him through it? How would I even tell him?

. . . my younger brother, a fixture of my whole life, and my mother and father, in their seventies and still going strong. I was their child. What could be worse than the death of one's child?

. . . my little passion, my writing, my "body of work"—a bunch of barely read pieces of fiction, a smattering of poetry, some pub-lished, some unpublished—leaving behind a miniscule trace in the world of who I was. At least I didn't have some unfinished magnum opus waiting vainly to be born.

. . . all the people I'd known, friends and co-workers past and present, those who changed me, made me, and the deep regret I felt that I didn't keep in touch with all of them, see their changes, know them really, so that I could say hello to them once again, and perhaps now goodbye.

And there was my job to face. The next day, I went to work. I had students to take care of. And what do you know? Stranger than fiction, irony of ironies, that week the focus of my class—the cho-sen theme of the academic English curriculum, the subject that would serve to galvanize language skills for my small group of international students—was cancer. All about cancer: types, causes, prevention, treatments, the search for a cure—a one-week mini-survey of this modern scourge.

At first I thought, no, I won't be able to handle it. I'll see my boss, let her know my situation and take at least some time off. In the back of my mind, too, was the thought of a more permanent leave, to focus on getting better or, if it came down to it, just liv-ing life in the time I had left. But I remembered something. I'd delivered the week's material before and recalled an inspiring NFB documentary by a Canadian filmmaker about his own struggle with a rare adrenal cancer. It was called *In My Own Time: Diary of a Cancer Patient.*

Joe Viszmeg was forty-two when he died in 1999. For eight years, since he was first diagnosed in 1991, the doctors kept telling him he had less than a year to live. His film chronicles the first four of those years. Watching it again with a new urgency, a couple of things stood out for me: one, his reaction to being suddenly confronted with his mortality, so that he was now thinking about his own death every five or ten minutes; as well, his feeling of being cheated by fate, with all the beauty in the world turning ugly, existing merely to rub salt in his wounds. An all-encompassing pall had fallen over him. For me, nobody was yet telling me how long I had left to live. But the feeling of being cheated was becoming real. Whereas once I envied the young, those in their twenties, say, just starting out in life, I was now finding myself looking at anyone "older" with a stewing bitterness, bitter that I might never see old age. Some of my colleagues had reached their fifties and beyond. I thought of Bridget. She'd seen that milestone. No longer could I think in relative terms, it seemed. Time had turned into a mercilessly linear, absolute thing.

Joe, however, repeatedly defied the doctor's prognosis. In time, what emerged for him was a much more positive and life-affirming understanding of his own limited powers. He describes a "paradox of reality," meaning the paradox of listening to the medical doctors, finding their assessment of his situation hard to refute, but, at the same time, being compelled to create a *new* reality, one that would ultimately deny theirs. To this end, he undertook a long and fruitful personal odyssey to seek out alternative therapies. As Joe explains, if Western medicine was going to write him off, he would write it off.

What Joe actually did was put Western medicine in perspective. He understood that medical doctors don't offer certainty. They can't tell if you are absolutely fine. They can't even tell how ill you really are. Truly knowing these states is conditional on the limited knowledge of science today, on averages, on probabilities extrapolated from empirical observation. Science doesn't see individual potential, nor is it able to account for some still pretty large unknowns. As Joe found out, health is much bigger than the physical presence or absence of a disease: Health is, rather, a troika "of mind, spirit, and body," a project the whole person undertakes through a lifetime.

And I would add something more. In the film we see Joe's wife, Rachel, ache with sadness for the isolating effect the diagnosis had on him. Also, Joe deeply regrets not telling his daughter earlier about his disease. He kept her in the dark because knowing would be too painful for her. "A big mistake," he says. Yes, it was—for the fourth essential of health is the support and understanding of others. Not a troika, then, but a quad, a square: mind, spirit, body—and a loving community.

Which brings me to my students. I began the weekly theme as I usually do, by encouraging them to tap into personal experience, to connect the stuff of their lives with an unfamiliar area of study, the better to create a desire to communicate in new ways in a new language. For this theme, I would have to be more delicate than usual, so I left it open, suggesting they were free to tell or not tell about any experience or contact they might have had with the disease. A Korean student mentioned his grandfather's death from lung cancer. A Chinese girl told us her mother was a Traditional Chinese Medicine practitioner who often treated cancer patients. They spoke honestly but with little engagement. Even within their own families, cancer seemed a distant thing. So I thought as I looked at their young faces, their lives filled more with dreams and possibilities than anything like endings. Then a powerful urge took hold of me, to spill it, to just say, "Well, guess what, you know something? I have cancer, cancer of the kidney. How about that? Any questions? I'll tell you everything I've learned so far." Of course, I did no such thing.

But the impulse told me of my need, a need that was getting stronger by the day. That is, to tell people, the world, what was happening to me, to plea for support, to create a community of understanding. At that point, my wife knew, but not my parents, my son, my brother, or anyone else. I felt I had to start telling people, and knew how hard it would be. Trust would be the measure of whom I could tell next, those who would want to know because they cared. I decided to visit my mother and father on the weekend.

I never got the chance.

On Friday afternoon, I was home early from the college. The sun was shining through our kitchen window. I was talking with my wife about how to break the news not only to my parents, but to our son as well. The phone rang. I recognized the voice of my urologist.

"This will be the best call you'll ever get in your life," he said. He'd looked at the CAT scan himself. "It isn't a cancer after all! Your tumour is benign. I confirmed it with the radiologist."

"Are you sure? Are you really sure?" I asked.

"Yes," he said. "I'm sure."

But was he really, really sure? He was wrong the first time, wasn't he? Doubt dampened my elation; anger, my relief. How could he be so positive, so definite? Here he was, giving me the certainty I'd wanted, and I couldn't accept it. Why the hell did they tell us anything if it might not be true?

I couldn't stay angry, though. It seems this benign tumour, called an angiomyolipoma, is quite rare, exceedingly so in men. The CAT scan revealed its fatty non-malignant features. Ten or so years of clinical experience had told the good doctor that kidney tumours in men were cancerous 99.9 percent of the time. I was a statistical anomaly. This explained the error. Yet, in the urologist's view, his judgement was entirely correct, according, that is, to his method. So were Joe Viszmeg's doctors not wrong in their regular one-year-to-live prognoses. Their professional judgement rests on the reasonable premises of science. Statistics equal averages and probabilities, not individuals.

You might now call me one lucky dude with a proverbial horse-shoe up my butt, and a good story to tell to boot. Okay. Still, I'd always taken Fortune as a fickle goddess who would as likely frown as smile. Why me? Why not me? "As flies to wanton boys, are we to the gods; they kill us for their sport," says the Bard. But if I were to take any lesson at all from Joe Viszmeg's film, this experience was not a matter of fortune at all, not something arbitrary and alien that merely happened to me. The benign tumour inside is just me, myself. It reveals who I am. It is part of the state of health I'm in according to my body and its interconnectedness with my mind, my spirit, and my community. The doctor told me I was sick. Then he told me I was fine. Which is it? Our individual lives are as much potential as reality, as much what could be as what is. We get no reports on the former, but that's where I believe we can seek and locate a missing dimension in the search for our whole selves.

Two things remain. The urologist cited a Mayo Clinic study that told him a six-centimetre benign mass in the kidney is a borderline case for treatment options. It's just small enough to leave alone, but if it grows any larger the risk of it bursting and bleeding out increases. Then it won't be so benign. But before that happens, a procedure, such as a surgery, would be warranted. On the other hand, it may simply shrink and waste away all on its own. As a result, I now have periodic CAT scans to monitor the tumour's activity. Am I safe or am I in danger? Am I fine or am I ill? We sit on the border, always in-between; it defines our existence, the ongoing project.

Then there's my original complaint: the pain in my abdomen. What's going on? Is the tumour the cause? No, my urologist says, it must be something else. He refers me to my GP: "For that, you're back to square one." Square one. Back to the beginning. One square with four points of light: mind, spirit, body, and community, always at the threshold of sickness and health. This place, where every day is square one, means potential, not hypochondria. I don't know if I'm really there yet, but it seems a better place to be and, if possible, remain, as I go forward. No matter what the doctors say.

Sailing into Seventy

Beverley A. Feather

I really can't recommend old age. Oh, I knew I'd get wrinkles and grey hair, but I imagined I'd handle all that with grace and hair dye. That part of aging didn't bother me. To be honest, it didn't thrill me, but I can live with such minor body changes, particularly now that I know they're just the tip of the iceberg.

The real knowledge that I was changing ages wasn't signalled by grey hair; in fact I viewed grey hair as an opportunity to finally see how I looked as a blonde. The first tremor in my serenity occurred when my friends and I all had our cholesterol shoot up and our thyroids slow way down. The body that had always worked so well was suddenly malfunctioning, and I'll admit I was a bit peeved and reluctant to become part of the medicated generation.

To add to the injustice, I had to start wearing glasses—and each year they got stronger and the printed directions on labels got smaller and smaller until I also had to invest in a magnifying glass.

It is extremely annoying the way the younger generations mumble. In my day we took elocution lessons. We knew how to enunciate and project. I thought I had at least trained my own children to speak clearly, but they, too, are becoming part of the mumbling masses. I tire of asking them to repeat what they've said and of following them around by the ear, so to speak, leaning way in with my good ear to catch what they are saying. Sometimes I just pretend to follow the conversation, nodding and smiling at what seem appropriate moments. Of course, if I miss an important detail and nod and smile when someone allegedly has asked, "Could you turn on the oven at two?" then they all raise their eyebrows behind my back, when obviously the problem lies in their sloppy speech.

The motto for the aging should be "Adjust, Adjust, Adjust." I failed to adjust or be graceful when I began to shed more hair than twelve cats during a hot spring; in fact, I became seriously pissed off with aging gracefully. Wrinkles did not bother me, but bald I could not handle. Rogaine nudged its way into my medicine cabinet, next to my medications for thyroid and cholesterol; and as my joints stiffened up a bit, flax oil, glucosamine chondroitin, and calcium claimed shelf space. Contrary to what ads and magazine articles might lead you to believe, vitamins have not cured all my ills. The dam continues to spring new leaks. My body is no longer as user-friendly as it once was. I can no longer take it for granted, and now I must check with my parts before leaping to my feet as a whole.

Some days it seems every part of me conspires to mutiny. My wardrobe still contains strappy three-inch heels. I keep them as mementoes of a past age—and truly some are approaching antique status. I can't quite remember when my feet began their campaign for orthopaedic inserts and sturdy lace-up shoes. It isn't just that high heels hurt, but my balance isn't what it once was either. It really isn't cool to fall off your shoes.

As if greying, balding, slowing, and stiffening isn't enough to contend with, there is the matter—grey matter—of the memory. This is the touchiest area of all. I definitely bristle when my memory is called into question. For a while I plotted to record every conversation with my adult children so there'd be no argument over my being right about who agreed to do what, when, or who had what, and where who put it. Unfortunately I keep forgetting my pocket tape recorder.

Privately, I realize that being busy and having important matters to think about means I don't always concentrate on the more mundane details, like where I put my purse or the keys, or when I was to pick up a family member. I realize others might not understand that my memory is not failing; I'm just preoccupied, so I use more Post-it notes and lists and appointment books and calendars. In fact, I now have a forest of reminders, if I could just remember to read them.

With age there also comes a loss of stature—literally. In the last ten or fifteen years I've grown down two-and-a-half inches. I birthed three children without a murmur, but when the nurse at the doctor's office proved to me that I had indeed shrunk, I will admit to letting out a wail heard in the parking lot. So much for coping gracefully. I've definitely crossed over to the Dylan Thomas "Rage, rage against the dying of the light" school of thought.

Somewhere around forty-five, I started a mental "to do before" list. Somewhere around fifty-five, I started editing the list. Items that involved being cold, wet, or sleeping on the ground began to disappear. Heck, without just the right mattress, I won't sleep in a bed anymore. My joints have become very particular about where I lay me down to rest.

Bungee jumping hasn't quite been crossed off the list, as I am pondering whether it might be a means of regaining an inch or so, but skydiving has been axed, along with other high-impact activities I might be unable to hobble away from. Who knew the activities at the local seniors' centre would begin to look interesting?

My bladder has gained a prominent position on my board of directors. In a power play it declared I had to remain within a half-hour radius of a bathroom. The bladder works better than electronic monitoring or house arrest. Being old demands one become crafty enough to outsmart such tyrants.

Invitations to long hikes or kayak trips demand sacrifice or great humility. Simply cutting out liquids for ten or so hours before a long outing can buy freedom, but while camels may be able to hike across vast hot deserts, going without water for days, the human body tends to rebel. Humility is the smarter but harder route. On long hikes I can usually count on a well-endowed bush without a bear behind it, but out on the ocean in a kayak I faced a dilemma that finally forced me to invest in those golden-age products such as Poise and Depends.

Nature, however, is contrary. While the bladder increases its activities, other functions become sluggish, and so high-fibre cereals replace my cornflakes, or I start the day the Metamucil way. While I kick-start my system with roughage, I now begin to read my morning paper backwards, starting at the end with the obituaries and working my way back to the less important details of the world news. I know people who count up those they have outlived like notches in their belts.

Social gatherings in my age group no longer begin with the marriage-birth-work exchange of news, but rather with the hospital-cemetery update. At my age you don't ask, "How are you?" unless you really mean it and have an hour to spare. A more apt name for the "Golden Years" might be the "Griping Years."

There are some lesser known facets of aging, and comparing gripes with older friends is an important source of information. For instance, what used to be automatic body reactions aren't anymore. I find I don't automatically swallow successfully anymore. Something goes awry every so often and I choke on my own spit, to put it indelicately. Without griping, I wouldn't have found out this happens to other people and was not the beginning of some frightening terminal condition.

Still, there are things to look forward to. My friend says she read that it's just as cheap to live on a cruise ship as it is in a rest home, and there is the added advantage of having a doctor right on the premises who will make cabin calls. Imagine travelling the world with people who clean, make your bed, and feed you gourmet meals. If they still allow burials at sea, this could become quite the package deal.

Smart cruise lines could even start a savings club towards living aboard. They could have "Sail Into Your Seventies" cruises for seniors only.

I've checked with all of my body parts and, so far, other than an advisory against too much rich food, it seems like a plan.

Ghosts

Jane Silcott

I sprained my knee last year in a ski accident, a middling sprain, with some cartilage damage that hasn't yet healed. I've had surgery. A year later, the knee is still weak. It bites at me sometimes, climbing stairs or with sudden movements. It is always a presence, a weak place I negotiate with.

Marni Jackson, in her book *Pain: The Fifth Vital Sign*, says that pain fuses the body and mind and that it is something like a river, pulling tributaries of older pains into the flow of fresh insult, so that a person stung by a bee, for instance (as she was, inspiring her to write the book), will remember and feel other pains, including emotional ones. I know that's true. Along with this pain and the visits to medical professionals has come a series of ghosts—old injuries and trails of ongoing grief that haunt me with their shades and chains.

The first and most persistent ghost is the one that tells me I'm accident-prone. It spoke up as soon as I felt my knee go and hasn't really shut up since. It's an irritating ghost because it's got a smug "gotcha" quality that makes my teeth grind. I think it got that way because I'd become cocky, thinking I'd learned how to manage this body/mind of mine after some fairly spectacular mistakes and that nothing so foolish would ever happen to me again. So it could also be called the ghost of arrogance and presumption, the ghost of a fool, the ghost of misguided belief.

At thirteen, I broke a leg. At nineteen, about three months after I'd dropped out of university and was living a confused wayward life at my parents' ski cabin north of Toronto, I hurtled down an icy downhill race course at about ninety kilometres per hour and hit the lip of a long rolling hiccup in the hill. For a few moments I rose in a pure line, like a vector in a math problem. When gravity caught up with me again—and the realization that my wild, airy ride would end badly—I noticed a man below me scurrying out of the way. First, I worried that I'd land on him. Then I worried that I'd spend the rest of my life in a wheelchair.

The wheelchair came true, but only for a month; for two months before that I lived on my back in hospital in a body cast, my left arm extended above me in a Statue of Liberty pose. The experience, though painful and sometimes terrifying, was also relatively easy. Compared to the confusion of living away from my parents for the first time with no clear structure or direction, it was a relief to have my life simplified. My job was to get better. No one expected anything else of me.

Last year I turned fifty. Marni Jackson says it's common for women to injure themselves on the cusp of menopause. While I bristle a little at finding myself part of a common trend, I also have to admit it makes sense. The knee injury happened during a wilderness cross-country ski trip with a friend who also turned fifty that year. If pressed, we might both have admitted we were on a "Let's prove we're not dead yet" mission.

There's no point pretending that going out into the wild is anything less than a test. The clever gadgets and bright clothing in the outdoor equipment stores make us feel as though we're in control, but when we get out there, when there's nothing but mountains and trees, when the trail markers are gone, the sky is a uniform grey and the wind is suddenly pressing into your face like a hand, you are alone with whatever mix of knowledge, experience, strength, and courage, or lack of it, that you bring.

The existentialists say our experiences make us who we are. At a conference on pain that Jackson attended, a neurobiologist said the memory of injury "reorganizes" the brain. When I flew in the downhill race, there was at first the marvellous surprise of air, and then there was a very long moment when I hung there before falling, still weightless. Is that moment part of who I am? Did all the injuries I sustained on landing reorganize my brain?

When I broke my leg at thirteen, I felt a thud and lay still, not in pain, but knowing something profound had happened. When I broke my pelvis, shoulder, and wrist in the downhill crash, there was the same absence of pain and sense of stillness. At the moment when my knee went, even though there was an ominous "pop" inside, the pain flashing like fire up to my hip was reassuring. Jackson says our bodies produce a natural opiate in extreme circumstances to help us survive, so a person whose arm is being chewed by a tiger, for instance, feels no pain and is able to think about how to escape. Not that a ski hill is populated by tigers, but it is remarkable how much thinking I've been able to do every time I've been injured. With the knee, though the pain was searing, and I knew I'd screwed up in a major way, I also knew I wouldn't require rescue. And although several ghosts clamoured gleefully around me, there was also another ghost: the one that emerges in the aftermath—the ghost of the good patient, the ghost of the survivor, the ghost of the person who needs to begin again (and again and again). Do I injure myself when things are too complicated? When I need confirmation that I matter to people? Or that I can do this one thing: get better?

One day in hospital when I was still in the body cast, a resident told me my pelvis had been shattered and that I'd never walk again. He sat on the edge of my bed to tell me this, as though, what? That the imposition of his body into my space—my fragile, fragile space—could comfort me? That night I woke up screaming. I had seen myself walking like the Hunchback of Notre Dame, my left leg slewing awkwardly beneath me. Was this the ghost of what might have been, or the ghost of how I saw myself then—an outsider, a girl who didn't know how to fit in?

Pain makes people doubt themselves, says Jackson. I agree. The longer the pain of this injury has lasted, the more I've doubted myself. I've doubted I was ever an athlete. I've doubted I would ever be one again. I've doubted my right to medical care. When a sports doctor told me I'd have to learn to live with it, I nearly burst into tears on his examining table. "Will it hurt anyone if I just go talk to the surgeon?" I asked him.

There are days when other ghosts walk through me. The sports doctor had kind eyes behind the strain—perhaps I recognized something in him; my father was a medical man too. When I was rolled into hospital in Toronto after my downhill crash, I heard a nurse say excitedly, "That's the dean's daughter"; then an authoritative voice said, "She'll be treated the same way as everyone else." I am always surprised when grief hits, when it comes into my body, inhabits me like a low-lying flu, a miasma of *sad*, until something releases it: someone's kindness or ignorance; a glimpse of an old man in a store wearing the same sort of hat that my father did; or a hand, my own, with age spots blooming just like his.

A knee is an intersection of bones and cartilage, a weight-bearing intersection, a hinge. Knees can be damaged with blows or hard twists, ligaments can tear, the cartilage can rip. In other parts of the body, blood would carry healing cells to the damaged area, but in knees, especially the inner core, there's no blood flow, so if there's a tear or crack or bruise, the healing is slow or nonexistent. An MRI showed a tear in my meniscus. My GP, who's known me for years, said, "Why haven't you had surgery yet?"

My knee in the camera's eye, from the interior view, is stunning. I'm Venus in there. The head of my femur is pale and glowing like a full moon on a clear night. "The head of your femur looks very nice," the surgeon agrees, his voice muffled by the poor quality of the video. Still, you can hear the slight lilt, his sure precise way of speaking, the syllables mulled over, like marbles. I'm sitting on the couch with my family, watching the tape of my surgery on our TV. The surgeon is moving around inside my knee with a camera, a rounded metal probe, and a small grinder that looks in profile like a set of shark's teeth. The tools have been inserted through metal tubes that enter my knee through three small incisions. On our TV, my muscle tissue is pink and bright, while the ligaments are thick white bands that glisten like the inside of an oyster shell. In the background, against a muscle wall, there's a small, darker red shape that looks like a flatfish. Along the edges, long feathered bits of white matter move in the currents of water that were pumped into the joint so the surgeon could see better. This is synovial matter, the surgeon says. It's normal. I think it looks like veils fluttering in the wind, one of them like an anemone with its feelers trailing out.

"Your meniscus looks fine," the surgeon says, pointing his probe at a yellowy disc with a perfect curving C-shaped edge. It looks like a communion wafer. "But your cartilage is damaged here. See these fissures?" He moves the probe over something that looks like cracks in old linoleum—when he presses, they open, like small crevasses. "Nothing we can do about that," he says, "but you have a lot of synovial matter." The shark teeth whir and the white bits fly past with small red curls of blood that look distinct at first, like tiny rivers, then diffuse into clouds.

Sometime later, cutting meat off the bone for soup, I recognize the joint and have to press my mind away from thinking of the red tissue under the knife as muscle like my own. I'm thinking vegetarianism, animal rights, the plastinated bodies I'd seen at the Body Worlds exhibit. The pig's bone looks beautiful too. I recognize ligament, feel its rubbery strength and study how it funnels into a furrow in the bone. I tug to see how firmly it's attached; then I pull the joint apart and find the plate of yellowish tissue, which must be the meniscus. I'm not able to investigate further—the flesh in front of me is too familiar, and I decide I've gone far enough. I quickly chop the meat into small pieces and consign the bone to the garbage, not letting myself think of the pig and its short and sturdy life.

After surgery, I visit the surgeon, who tells me the cartilage under my kneecap had been bruised in my fall and that it was most likely the cause of my pain. There was nothing much he'd done in the operation to help that, he added, then told me it would heal of its own accord in about two years. "So, was it worth going in?" I ask, afraid I might offend him with this question—afraid, too, of his answer.

"Now we know how to treat it," he says. "Now we know exactly what is wrong with it."

Jackson says, "It's better to have pain that has a name than to suffer something wordless." Do I feel better knowing the name for my pain is "bruise"?

I limp away, thinking about pain and words and the way I hurl myself against mountains every time I face some shift in my life. When my children were young, they threw tantrums at any change. Leaving our house to go to a friend's, then leaving the friend's, they'd throw themselves on the floor and howl. I'd have to pick them up and carry them out under my arms, their furious bodies squirming against mine.

At my daughter's elementary school I pick up a hand-drawn sign that's fallen on the floor and put it back on the wall. "Self Control," it says. "I find I'm saying that one more and more," the teacher walking beside me comments, and then we both look at each other and laugh: two middle-aged women, our voices redolent with ghosts.

Chicken for Six

Kim Clark

I'm in the MS Clinic out at the university. I'm trying to think about neurological questions for my doc but drift away into dinner preparations for tonight. I've done what I can. It feels like this morning was a long time ago, and my highly acclaimed Chicken in Mourning dish is veiled in truffles in the fridge at home, waiting for me and my potluck friends. I can't really focus on that either.

Then, as I sit there, I remember going to this same MS Clinic for my annual check-up a few years after I was allowed to have an official MRI name for my condition. I was shocked when I walked into the waiting room. Most folks here were older, parked between semi-animate caregivers, wheelchairs, metal walkers—a constrained herd huddled near the magazine rack. I thought *good*, no young ones here struggling to be able. Then I thought *bad*, me having to deal with this unpredictable disease so many more years.

No receptionist at her welcome post. I sat down next to the wrinkled, anxious faces, partnered with their weary mates. Anxiety. Wow, I thought, there's a lot I don't know about MS.

When the receptionist showed up, I headed back to the counter. I felt all those waiting faces swing in curious unison to watch my territorial negotiations, eyeballs glued across my back, an unusual response from other disabled folks. If I could have jerked my head around fast without falling, I'd have given them the look.

"Can I help you?" name-tagged Mary asked.

"I have an appointment with Dr. Sharni for two o'clock."

"Dr Sharni? For the MS Clinic?"

"Yes. That's right." A swipe of uncertainty. Shit. What now? Don't tell me he's not here, I thought.

"He's not here," Mary said. "I mean, this isn't the MS Clinic."

"What do you mean? This *is* the MS Clinic. This is where I always come. Has it moved?"

There was something I wasn't getting. I could no longer trust name-tagged Mary. I felt a flush. I was pinking up like Mary's lipstick. The eyes on my back were becoming downright intrusive.

"I know I've been here."

Maybe my reality wasn't a shared one. Uncooperatively solipsistic. I was losing my mind. Maybe I should have gotten down on my hands and knees right there, right then, and looked for it under the counter, because it sure as hell felt like it had shrunken to the size of a peppercorn and fallen out my ear and rolled far, far away.

"Usually," said Mary, "but it's Tuesday."

I wanted to scream, "AND YOUR POINT BEING?"

But she, oh so complacently, went on to explain, "Today is the Alzheimer's Clinic. We share the space on alternate days. Are you sure it's not the Alzheimer's you wanted?"

WANT, Mary dearest? I was dumb. Relieved, somehow, to have survived the conversation, but dumb. Disorganized. Stupid. Forgetful. Wait a minute, no. I was annoyed. Mad. Pissed off. Somebody screwed it up, told me the wrong day.

"There must be some mistake." I dug in my purse for my official little reminder card, something I did strangely trust, as if a specific combination of symbols could erase every other identity, mistaken or not, from that waiting room. There was a mistake. Yeah . . . mine.

"Oh," I said. And I tried to walk out with some sort of dignity, but I seemed to have forgotten that too. Now the waiting room scene took on meaning—some were agitated because they didn't understand. Others, anxious because they did. Maybe I really did belong to the waiting room herd, the Alzheimer's Clinic, I thought. Thought seriously. Then hysterically, as I walked past the sign in the lobby, "Alzheimer's Clinic today."

I am really lucky, I thought. I only have the MS mess.

"Kim?" I'm back in the present, my Alzheimer's reverie broken. I hear my name, look up, and there he is. The compassionate, quietly smiling Dr. Sharni, always a blue shirt, navy tie. This is one of those places I never cry. It's my rule, my role here, and I am good. I follow him down the hall to his office. The guy always makes me feel like I'm part of a special club. He knows my history, my medical cartography, confessed personal interests from my chart, but he's so smooth that I can pretend that he remembers me from last year. That I stand out and maybe I do because I can still stand at all.

"So, Kim, you're looking well. How are things? Still writing? Going to school?" he asks, settling back in his swivel chair for a comfy chat. I want to hug him. Squeeze him in his comfy swivel chair. Let him pat my back while I tell him how good everything is.

And I verbally comply, almost at ease but trying to keep my adrenaline up so I can show him, prove to him that I am no worse. "Great, actually. Yeah, I'm still writing. Not so much schooling." Dropped my courses, but won't go there with Dr. Sharni today. Too openly stressful. Sign of dysfunction. "Not much change physically. I've needed the cane, like, I haven't been able to do without it at all in the last year." But I'm quick to reassure him before he drops his compassionate chin. "Actually some things are better." I fail to mention I'm living on my own now. Retain information control. Reticent disclosure. He assumes I mean physically and I let him be right.

"Well, good. Let's take a walk then," says Dr. Sharni. This is my cue. The performance. He stands in the doorway (upstage left), holding my cane, watching me progress, veer, careen all the way down the carpeted hall (downstage), trying to ignore, hide, overpower my progressive disease and choking down my embarrassment at the failures of my body. He meets me with my cane before I'm halfway back, and I know that's not a good sign. (No applause, either.) But he says an upbeat "Uh-huh" before we head back into his office—he, to his notes, my file, my life now; me, to the exam table. I know this routine. Don't need prompts.

I lounge against the table, bracing myself for the fear-factor-trust-test. It's a lot like those team exercises where you let your trusting self fall back into the arms of your sincerely waiting teammates. Only this time I don't have to consciously fall back. I only have to stand still and close my eyes. The falling happens without my knowing. I can't tell I'm moving through air until my only teammate, Dr. Sharni, grips my arms to stop me and my eyes fly open, recognizing the magnitude of this flaw. I survive. Get control. Slow my heart, not from the feeling of falling but from the lack of it. Without my eyes I am incapable of erection—not *an* erection, for gawd's sake, but uprightness.

"Mm-hmm," my teammate doctor acknowledges, then notates, and motions me onto the table. I get rid of my shoes, climb up, swing my legs, while he writes more illegible notes, data, information, in-formation, about deformed me.

We move into the second act. This is the least uncomfortable but the most difficult, not physically, but because the touch of his fingers brushing, stroking my cheeks so softly, brings up an ache of longing, the magnitude almost insurmountable.

He asks, "How's the sensation here? Anything different?" I want to draw his fingers into my mouth with my tongue. It is that bad, this evocation, the slightness of touch. But I don't of course. I follow the script. Keep my tongue in my mouth, my thoughts in my head, saying, "No change."

Then, "Cover one eye. Follow my finger," he says, and my eyes, one at a time, follow as dutifully as they can. Then, taking my right hand, he places it near his shoulder, but instead of asking me to dance, he lets go, saying, "Okay, touch your nose." This sounds too easy and it is, but wait. When I switch to my left, the difficulty is always ridiculously beyond belief—a scary hesitation, my digit searching its memory bank for placement. The index finger on my left hand has forgotten where my nose is. How is that even possible? Somewhere between my brain and the tip of my finger, the memory of myself has been disconnected, the distance skewed, proprioception defiled.

Then he taps my elbows, knees, for reflex. The "bad" side is always a fascination. It seems logical to me that there would be little response along with little feeling, numb tingling, but in fact, the left knee flings up the lower leg with such ferocity it could be detrimental to Dr. Sharni if he were less wary, more weary.

We go through all the strength tests. In various positions I pull, he pushes, or he pulls and I push. And I play hard to prove I still can. He does the "Babinsky." This is the creepy one where he scrapes a stick or a key up the bottom of my foot, heel to toe. Nothing to do with dancing, but it does give the foot a certain newborn curl.

Then we move into the sharpie challenges. He pokes my extremities repeatedly with a long pin. I respond with "Sharp" or "Pressure" unless I can't feel it at all, in which case I remain mute, wondering what the hell is taking him so long to find a good sharp place.

"There is some improvement in isolated areas, actually. Your fingers. That's great!" he says, adding notes to my file. I haven't succeeded in totally pleasing him, though.

"Enough to slide me down the scale?" I ask, knowing I was a five out of ten. I'm talking about the Krutzky Disability Status Scale. I hate this scale, this code, this cipher, but always ask. Need to know. Did I change? I want a better number. I want to be luckier. I want to be less, like maybe a one.

"No. Sorry, Kim. Other areas haven't done quite as well. Your gait, more spasticity. You're bordering on six. But it's minimal."

"So I'm even closer to ten than zero." Closer to death than symptom-free. Closer to death by MS. Death by chocolate would be more satisfying. In fact, I'm at six points, more than half-the-freakin'-scale away from where I was ten years ago. This is always a sobering moment. The one I want to handle well. Why do I always ask?

"Hmm. Five felt better." It's as close as I can get to acknowledgement.

"I know," he says, always gently. "But six is a huge area on this particular scale. Anyway, we know the scale is flawed. Just, well, no one's come up with a better way of measuring disability. It's difficult to knit together all eight neuro-systems."

I try to remember the flawed list. Eight, I think. *Cerebral. Visual. Cerebellar.* That sounds like a Jellicle from the musical *Cats.* My poetic mind shifts into gear while Dr. Compassionate Sharni writes up my life file. *Brainstem.* Reminds me of gardening. I wanted to grow Graceful, row after row of it in my garden, an abundance of Brainflowers on fragile stems against the porch steps at my feet.

TALES OF ILLNESS & RECOVERY

Damn. What were the others? Oh, yeah. *Pyramidal. Bowel and bladder.* How could I forget that one? *Sensory.* Sensual, sexual.

"Things seem really good. The progression is very slow." He has that ever-optimistic tone in his positive voice, so I'll follow his lead, relieved, put an up-look on my face, thinking, so this is progress. I am my own miniscule world, somehow killing itself.

"Any new studies I might fit into?" I need to keep myself up and open. I've been pretty game so far. Tried the steroids, a few different drugs, a few hundred injections. Hell, I even tried rubbing ostrich oil into my skin, but I got tired of smelling like turkey dinner. Kitty loved it though. We—Dr. Sharni and I remain a team—just haven't found the perfect potion yet. Scorpion venom is the latest thing. I read that it was the new high in Hong Kong, not an MS blocker. Maybe not a bad thing. "Scorpion venom might be more fun than the bee-sting therapy."

Dr. Sharni just smiles and says, "I think you've pretty much had a chance at every therapy we've got so far."

"What about the one that's all over the news right now?"

"You're not naïve to treatment with this drug, which makes you ineligible for the study. You've already tried it with a much lower dose. I'll make sure and let you know though, if anything promising comes up. Research is ongoing."

I admit I'm not naïve or virginal or anything remotely pristine, even with protocol pharmaceuticals. I've been around the block with a few drugs. But I'm already at six.

He goes on, "And there is improvement in bladder function and finger strength without any medication. Any change in libido? According to your file, you've had a pretty inactive or lost sex drive for quite some time, since the onset really. It's common with MS. We've talked about it."

I keep a straight face while I consider this for all of ten seconds.

That lovely lost libido was found during the last few months. In fact, it was never lost. Just subdued, suffocated, hidden, and nothing to do with MS, although I believed that was the cause for years. "No. No change," I lie, head bent, struggling into my shoes.

Dr. Sharni carries on. "If you're worried about any of this at some point, want to talk to someone, we can line up an appointment with Ruth, the psychologist here. I think you've met with her before." Of course he'd remember my mental crash-and-burn fiasco.

"I don't think I need to see a psychologist. Ruth . . . right. Rhymes with truth."

"Right," he says with a quiet laugh, trying to take this to a lighter level. I can feel my time's almost up. My turn's over. "Okay, then," he reassures me, pushing himself easily up to standing, and I manage to do the same.

"Anyway," I go on, "I'm relieved it's nothing worse, and the cane . . . well, I'm almost used to needing it."

"You manage just fine with it. And they are working on the research. Something may come up." Dr. Sharni sees me to the door, resting his hand against my shoulder blade. "Keep in touch."

"Thanks." Why do I always say thanks, no matter what?

"See you in a year." What a weird relationship. *Keep in touch.*

It's the "touch" word that sticks with me as I weave back out through the waiting room and finally to the sanctuary of my car. My comforting old car. Van, really, but I call it a "car" to piss off touchy automophiles. Touchy. *Touch.* But as I pull into heavy traffic, the word I can't shake is "six."

By the time I get home from the MS Clinic, park my car-sanctuary-van, pick up the soggy newspaper and get in the door, I'm MS-exhausted. I'll have a drink or six. Six. I'll put my feet up, even the good one. I carry the wine bottle under my arm, my favourite glass in hand, the orange one, the biggest, and the corkscrew in my pocket. *Settle down*, I think, as I flop backward into the couch.

The latent stress of post-clinic reality strangles me. The thought of people, guests, overwhelms me. It's too late to pull out, call off the dinner. These friends would understand, but stubborn pride demands another performance. I don't really want to be alone anyway. I know myself at least that well. I always resort to sorting my life out in a crowd. Takes the edge off.

I need to concentrate. I have an hour. One hour. Why did I think I could do this dinner easily? Breezily even? My chicken widow is still mourning in the fridge. The guests are coming about six. Six. "Let it go," I warn myself out loud, feeling powerless. It's just that I can't control someone else's restrictive number. I'll make it mine—the number six. Take it over. Take it on.

Focus is the issue. I'll go and clear off the table, get slowly busy. Occupied. Preoccupied. Let's see. We need all six chairs. Six. The microwave reads 5:36 when I hear the doorbell, but people are always ringing the doorbell here, so I wait till I hear voices. Voices that I recognize. Jackie's got a key. So I don't have to get up in case I can't. Why is she always early? I think it's an anti-social personality flaw. Goes against the grain, the chaff. Chafes me.

"Come on in," I call vaguely toward the door. The decision to cancel is out of my bitter hands. No mourning. No chickening out. It'll be great. Good, at least. It always is. I'll get seriously cheery. It's either buck up or fuck up—both of which I've had considerable experience with. I'll go with the former. Form the mood. Shape the evening. Even consider sharing the load.

Seeing It Through

Denise Halpern

Alone on the stage. No set. No props. Not even an audience. Alone on the stage and nobody's watching. What freedom this is. What a relief. I'd always felt that someone was watching me, assessing how I was doing: How successful am I in my career? How good am I at being a mother, a partner, a daughter, a friend? How clean is my house? How often do I change the sheets on my son's bed?

I'm too embarrassed to say. Okay . . . Once a month. Maybe. Look, there are all these tiny microscopic bugs that live in sheets, and the less you wash them, the more there are. So when my beautiful little boy slips his vulnerable body into his sheets, he's literally swimming in waves of disgusting little bugs. I know. I know they aren't hurting him. He probably doesn't even know they exist. It's all a mother's guilt. Why the guilt? Because we're being watched. And judged.

Or so I thought. But the thing is, we're not, it turns out. Each one of us is alone on the stage. And nobody's watching. This is real life. This is what's true. You remember when we were teenagers? And we thought people were looking at us all the time? And how often do you look in a mirror and try to see how others see you? You know you can't. You never can. Why? Because they don't see *you*.

I know, I know—here I am, after all. If you can't see me then who in the world are you looking at? Well . . . you don't see me. We can't really see each other. Each of us can only see through our own perceptions. Know what I mean? I am a different person to you than I am to anyone else. You see me through whatever else you have in this moment, and that includes what you decide to keep from other moments. Your history of perceiving me makes me who I am to you. You see?

Yeah, I know, we both see similar objects around us. Like you, I can see the nurse over there, and my IV pole, those flowers on the windowsill. Irises, I think. Lilies. I dunno. Anyway, my point is, I'm lying here, with all these tubes stuck in me, nobody telling me anything, getting really scared . . . And I think, what am I really scared of? Dying? And I find out that I'm not scared of dying. I'm scared of leaving my kid, and my partner, and my mom—all the people who depend on me, who need me, who I'm responsible for. What'll they do without me? How can I leave my son? The thought of his sadness crushes me. Man, we miss each other after being apart for a few days! A lifetime . . . that's unthinkable.

But then, right after I imagine the scenario—this scene in the future without me in it—it's like I hear a little voice in my head. I dunno. Maybe it's the drugs. Doesn't matter. The voice says, *They'll be okay.* They'll be okay.

See? I know they have their own lives. I have mine. That's the thing. The big revelation. This is my life. *My* life. I'm not living for them—I can't. I'm not responsible for them, as much as it seems like I am. That's me doing that. And the need thing. Do they really need me? Or is that just me again. They'll be okay. They have their lives, with their own stuff happening in them. I'm in each of their lives in the way that each of them has me in it. I can't know how it is for them. Not really.

Each of them, everyone, is on their own stage—we all are—

whether we're playing the lead or whatever part we want; we're choosing the cast; we're creating the sets, the props, the script, changing things around now and then, trying to get it right. You're doing what you want. You're the director. It's your play. And all the other actors? Of course, they're who you want them to be. You give them their roles.

Now you wonder just how you can be in so many places at once, right?—your own play, mine, everybody else's? You're not. *You're only in your own play.* That's the thing. There's really no one else on stage with you.

Just you. Alone on the stage. No set. No props. Not even an audience. Alone on the stage and nobody's watching. I'm all by myself. There's no audience. Nobody's watching. I can do whatever I want. I am free to do whatever I want. This is my life. My life.

The Bone Identity

Bonnie Bowman

This is what I do: I smoke. I drink. I sit on my ass. This is what I don't do: Take vitamins. Work out. Go to bed early. Am I ashamed of this? No. Am I proud of this? No. These are merely the facts. You need to know the facts.

Throughout my twenties, thirties, and forties, this dubious lifestyle has served me well. I have always embraced the motto, "If it ain't broke, don't fix it." Maintenance? I scoff.

Indeed, I have always taken some pride in being a low-maintenance gal, which, in itself, is a type of hubris I suppose. Doctors? I am loath to attend, even after I do a face-plant onto a sidewalk and discover upon awakening the next day that I've split my upper lip open, which, overnight, has morphed into a perfect square scab of black blood. I look like Hitler for two weeks until the scab falls off. When it does, I am left with a vertical scar, and until it fades, I bear a remarkable resemblance to Joaquin Phoenix. But worse, my pratfall has also bent my right thumb backwards. The pain of this is excruciating. I suffer in masochistic silence. I splint it myself with sticks and duct tape. I can't hold the weight of a beer glass and am forced to drink with my left hand for a month. When I remove the splint and realize I can no longer bend my thumb at all, thanks to my nifty splint job, I sigh and move on. I begin a rigorous training routine for my previously ineffectual left hand so that I can continue performing insignificant yet necessary tasks like opening jars.

When someone playfully pushes me one day and I split my eyebrow open on the corner of a couch, I do not go to the hospital, despite the ominous bloodletting. I let it heal on its own and am satisfied the resulting scar is less noticeable than if I had gotten stitches. The fact that I can still feel couch fibres permanently knotted up under my skin is of no consequence.

Where does this attitude come from? I like to think it's genetic. Maybe from my uncle Carl who lived out his days in the northern Ontario bush, who refused to see doctors in town, who accidentally chopped off his toe with an axe and cauterized it himself. Who, in his dotage, lived in the root cellar, literally choking to death on fumes from an ill-ventilated wood stove, while he spent his time building violins and writing his memoirs on paper he made himself from his own trees, then binding them in books made from tanned moose hide and sinews. Even as a child, I always thought my uncle Carl was a romantic, larger-than-life figure. I aspired to and adopted his fierce sense of independence and do-it-yourself philosophy. It is my birthright.

Truly, I come from hardy pioneer stock. Longevity runs in my family on both sides, my paternal great-grandmother living to be over a hundred years old, finally expiring alone in her own crooked house with no witnesses except her blind Pekingese dog and a million mice. Her daughter, my grandmother, lived well into her nineties, as did most of my relatives. The elderly among us who are still alive are easily cruising towards the century mark. In fact, the only people who died off early were those who had married into the family. This begs the supposition that either my relatives always married people from inferior genetic pools, or my relatives are all a bunch of murderers.

Armed with their unassailable genes, I breeze through life, knowing I'm fortunate. Knowing it's the luck of the DNA draw. I handily ignore the fact that all these hardy souls from whence I sprung did not smoke, did not drink, and definitely did not sit on their asses all day. If I do think about it, I figure my bad habits will cut maybe ten years off my expected inheritance of a lifespan, and I'll still outlive the majority of the population. This is not to say I'm not cognizant of the fact that something will go wrong eventually, that I could spend the last twenty years of my life smoking through a hole in my throat. For instance, somewhere along the way, I'm convinced I will need a quadruple bypass operation. I'm resigned to it.

Cloaked in my protective force field of heredity, I carry on. Smoking. Drinking. Sitting on my ass. And the inevitable bypass? Well, whatever. I get the bypass and life goes on and on. There are better things to do than worry about it. I should point out that this laissez-faire attitude concerning my outer shell is not blind bravado, not latent youthful conviction of immortality. This is fully realized. I've spent years working for doctors and am better informed than most lay people of the limitations and unexpected fuck-ups of this mortal coil that gradually strangles us to death. I am quite aware that the "it'll never happen to me" line of thinking is gonna bite you in the ass. Getting old sucks. I know this. Getting a bypass will suck. Getting uglier by the minute sucks. In fact, I've had arguments with other fiftyish women who rave about how they "love" getting older, à la "I love the age I'm at now." "I'm so much wiser." "I've never been happier." "I'm settled. I'm peaceful." Settled? Peaceful? That's the kiss of death right there. And by the way, Miss I'm-Happy-I'm-Getting-Older . . . are you even *in* menopause yet? Yeah, didn't think so. Talk to me when your bed has become a swamp and you're waking up ten times a night to take a piss. You'll be the first person in line for hormone replacement therapy, gobbling it up like candy. From there, you'll march straight to the plastic surgeon for your facelift. Why? Because you're so damn happy getting old, I guess.

Although my fortunate genetic make-up may prolong my lifespan well beyond what my lifestyle deserves, it does not preclude the growing horror of growing horribly older. Big things aside—like the top two on the hit list, cancer and heart disease—it's the little insidious events that rankle most. The inexorable disintegration of random parts of your body that you never gave much thought to. Your knee hurts when you crouch down and stand up. It takes longer to stand up. You lie in bed at night and your hips inexplicably ache. Hip replacement? God. Should I take calcium? Nah, I'll just eat more cheese. You suddenly need reading glasses. A crime, especially when most of your life is spent reading and/or writing while you sit on your ass and smoke and drink. Widening of your torso. Sagging of your jowls. Eggs committing mass suicide. Aches and pains. Limitations. All a precursor to encroaching immobility requiring possible body-part replacements, none of which are aesthetically motivated, all prosthetically motivated.

Which brings us to my own impending prosthetic replacements. I'm getting implants this year. No, not *those* implants. Dental implants. A couple of fake teeth, as opposed to a couple of fake tits. Apparently, unbeknownst to me, I've been experiencing gradual and steady bone loss in my mouth, this nasty bit of business happening unobserved way up under my gums. This is a very surprising and unexpected turn of events. My entire existence, I've been blessed with perfect teeth. Orthodontically correct. Completely cavity-free. The kind of teeth dentists have orgasms over. Now I'm set to lose a couple of the faithful chompers, thanks to freakish degenerating bone. Nothing spells "old" better than being toothless, I say. Of all the things I could have predicted going wrong with my body—and there are many—my perfect teeth never occurred to me. But in the last year or so, I've been noticing definite signs of wobbling in some of my upper teeth. Wobbling! What the hell? This is not something I can fix with duct tape.

Settled in the periodontist's chair, while he studies my X-rays with ill-concealed dismay, I ask, "So, what causes this bone loss anyway?"

I brace myself for the smoking lecture. In my experience with medical professionals, they seize every available opportunity to blast you with the smoking diatribe, because we might not realize that ingesting acrid cyanide-laced smoke into our lungs could be bad for our health. They are driven to lecture, obsessed with it. You've got a rash? "Stop smoking." You've got an axe sticking out of your head? "Stop smoking."

But the good Dr. K doesn't lay into me about smoking, which immediately endears him to me for life. The cause, or causes, could be many things, he says. Smoking is one of them (naturally). Menopause is another one (no surprise there, menopause causes everything). And here's the kicker. It could also be hereditary. Say it ain't so, doc!

Could be one of the above, or all of the above, or none of the above, he says. He shrugs. He doesn't know, he doesn't care. He just wants to fix it. It is his mission in life to save my perfect teeth. I love him.

Thus, I undergo the knife. The first, but likely not the last, shoring up of bodily disintegration. First order of business: bone grafting—the hope being to encourage new bone growth and sta-bilize some sketchy teeth. Growing additional bone will also be extremely helpful for the drilling and screwing of an implant into my head, because without a good bone base, we come perilously close to puncturing my sinus. As the doctor and I sit shoulder-to-shoulder and study the X-rays together like amiable colleagues, he points out my sinus. To an untrained eye, it looks like we've got no bone whatsoever to work with. It looks like my sinus is riding on my teeth roots.

"I think we've got enough room," muses Dr. K, tilting his head and squinting. He amends this assessment: "Barely."

And even if we don't, all is not lost, he assures me. He carelessly tosses off the option of sinus surgery. I blanch at the thought. We can sling my sinus up in some sort of hammock and keep it away from the drilling of the implant. Any hesitation I had entertained about bone grafting pales when compared to the thought of a sinus hammock.

Bring on the bone grafts, I say. Let's grow us some bone!

The procedure is onerous. The slicing and trimming and peeling up of gums is involved. Two hours to do but half your mouth. Bits of gum are hacked right off, exposing previously hidden parts of teeth. When it's done, I am sporting new gaps between my teeth up near the gum line, big enough to drive a truck through. My gums have been pushed up significantly, making me officially "long in the tooth." Thankfully, Dr. K leaves the gumline over my front teeth pretty much alone for vanity reasons, otherwise my smile would rival that of The Joker and strike fear into the hearts of small children—which, come to think of it, may not be a bad thing.

I bear the grafting trauma stoically, like I bear everything. I have a very high pain tolerance. I do not partake of the Valium that's offered me, which proves, if nothing else, I'm not a drug addict. I'd probably have kicked ass during labour if I had wanted kids (which I didn't), so I guess we'll never know about my mute expulsive efforts on that front.

As I stare up at the good doctor while he rips my face open and sings along to the radio through his mask, I mumble, "Where do you get the bone from?" Or, more accurately, "Eh oo ew geh uh oh um?"

Cows.

I digest this unsettling bit of news, I chew the information like cud. When we're done with the first two-hour session, I sit dazed in the chair, drooling bloody saliva onto my bib, and express my shock and awe at the fact that I now have cow bone in my rapidly swelling mouth. What about mad cow disease, I splutter. Hoof and mouth!

He smiles tolerantly at me. He explains about it being synthesized. He tells me the cows might save a few teeth that would otherwise be history. He says it's safe. He says we'll know in a year if the bone grafting "took." He has high hopes for my mouth. I love him again.

Many months and several procedures later, I am now minus one upper eyetooth—a fang, as it were. For the time being, pre-implant surgery, I have a removable fake tooth to replace it. They call it a "flipper" for some inexplicable reason. I hate my fake tooth, even though it looks just like the real deal, stained to be an exact match with the rest of my teeth—a clever tint from the fabulous du Maurier collection no doubt. The fake tooth has a pink plastic partial palate attached to it, which is a terrible thing. I can't taste food as well as I should. I have a lisp. My tongue doesn't know what to do with it. I am told my tongue will train itself to the alien presence, but I don't want to train my tongue. Ergo, I seldom wear my four-hundred-dollar fake fang and opt instead for a hillbilly grin that might look rakishly charming on a twenty-year-old, but verges on scary with someone of my advancing hag-years. Nonetheless, I eschew the wearing of it entirely, unless I have to make an impression on somebody, which also, it should be noted, is an occasion that happens less and less the older you get. I have newfound respect for people who wear full dentures. I nag everybody I know to floss like fiends. I spend hours picking crap out of my perfect teeth.

Granted, this experience doesn't come close to losing a limb, or undergoing chemo, or getting a colostomy, or a heart transplant. But it is an eye-opener. I'm losing bone. Bone is not a good thing to lose. Bone keeps everything hanging on; without it, things fall out. Useful things like teeth. All those nightmares about my teeth crumbling and falling out—those nightmares we all apparently experience—guess what? They're true.

As I stand in front of my bathroom mirror one day, selecting various pointy instruments from my recently acquired dental booty and raking them between my teeth before brushing with my new Sensodyne toothpaste and gargling with antiseptic mouth-wash, it suddenly occurs to me that this is not the first time I've been made aware of having bone loss. Years ago, I was told my neck was crumbling away. Cervical vertebrae, C4 to C7, or some-where thereabouts. Disc degeneration. CAT scans, X-rays, MRIs—all told the gruesome tale. Aside from chronic neck pain, which I had blithely attributed to being hunched over a computer for years—and naturally, did not consult a doctor about—I ignored it. That is, I ignored it until the day I woke up with tunnel vision and felt really, really stoned and not in a good way. Also, I was not able to walk properly and kept tripping over my feet (see aforemen-tioned falling episodes). Freaked out, I floated into my GP's office from whence I was immediately shipped off to a top neurologist who, it so happened, was in a wheelchair, which, frankly, didn't inspire much confidence. My bizarre symptom complex had raised the spectre of multiple sclerosis, and nobody was dicking around with that possibility. There were sidelong worried glances between the medical professionals that did not escape my notice. Fortunately, after a battery of tests, it was discovered I did not have MS, merely chronic degeneration of cervical discs. There is nothing to be done about this, until my head falls off.

Having cannily made the connection between my vanishing verte-brae and disappearing dental bone, I decided to do something I seldom do: ask my mother for her opinion. I was curious to see if this type of rot is infecting other branches of the family tree. I hoped it was, because then I could blame the family genes and continue smoking with impunity. I began with the neck thing. My mother's response?

"Oh yes, all the women in our family have it," she replied breezily, reeling off aunts and cousins and including herself in the list of bobble-headed relations.

Excellent news. I light up a smoke.

The dental thing was a little harder to pin down because apparently in the "old days," if you had any type of ailment at all, the wisdom of the times was to have all your teeth pulled out of your head. Teeth were considered the root of all evil. All manner of viruses and bacteria and other nefarious infiltrators were believed to enter your body and wreak havoc via your mouth. If you wanted to play it safe, you pulled all of the offending teeth. My maternal grandmother, my mother said, had some kind of flu-like bug, and they yanked all her teeth out at once, when she was barely forty years old.

"They were all good teeth too," my mother hissed. "She had perfect teeth, like you do."

When I inquired further, asking specifically about Uncle Carl, I was told he extracted all his own teeth long before he was considered old. If he got a toothache, out came the trusty pliers. I beam with pride at this nugget. In fact, all the northern relatives were likely toothless before their time, whether they needed it or not. My parents, on the other hand, still have all their original teeth. They attribute this to fleeing the bush, seeing dentists regularly, and drinking fluoride-laden City of Toronto tap water. Good for them. Maybe my big mistake was fleeing Toronto and drinking Vancouver tap water for twenty-four years. No matter. I'm back in Toronto again with my new best friend, Dr. K, who will save me from a lifetime of being indentured.

In the meantime, I go for regular three-month check-ups and enforced deep-root cleanings. Together, Dr. K and I check the mobility/stability of my teeth. The good doctor is pleased with my progress and I bask in his praise. Things have tightened up already, he says with satisfaction, which is refreshing since it's the only place on my body where things are actually tightening up. From the state of my mouth pre-periodontist, there were four or five questionable teeth. Now, at least for the time being, there are only two. One is already history. We're just waiting for the one beside it to wobble right out of my skull or otherwise cause some sort of problem before we start screwing around with replacement options. I asked him once if I could get gold teeth, expecting some eye-rolling, as if I were a teenager pushing the bounds of propriety merely to provoke a reaction. But again, he surprised me. Sure, you can get gold teeth if you want, he said, not batting an eye. You can get whatever you want. You can get a diamond in your tooth if you like. Apparently this is not an uncommon request nowadays, thanks to rappers. But the fact that he was completely amenable to a fifty-one-year-old menopausal white chick getting gold teeth, without trying to dissuade me from such a rash course of action, made me not want them as much. Did I mention I love him? That said, possessing a gold fang does have some weird sort of allure for me. I feel like I'd be embracing my defects, rather than hiding them behind look-alike replacement parts, as if I were ashamed of my growing decrepitude.

Don't get me wrong—there may be no shame, but I'm clearly not thrilled that my teeth are falling out. It is a bit of a shock, more so than the other obvious signs of aging, like greying hair, loss of muscle tone, and wrinkling up. Those I expected. And despite their devolving natures, I still have hair, muscles, and skin. My fang, however, sits in a ring box. Every now and then, I take it out and gaze at it wistfully. It's huge. It's no longer in my mouth. And it's soon to be joined by its disagreeable neighbour, at which point the gap in my smile will be too wide to ignore and will considerably hamper any eating efforts. As I put the fang back in its box, I consider making the beginnings of a voodoo tooth necklace. Or maybe if I become a super-famous author I can sell my teeth on eBay to pay for the implants. But whatever I do, I can't seem to bring myself to simply throw my tooth in the garbage. This tooth, after all, is the first piece of my body that has been removed due to degeneration. I still have my tonsils, my appendix, all of my essential organs, my limbs, and what's left of my brain. And although many people seem to manage quite nicely with no teeth whatsoever, I think I'd rather not.

As an ironic aside to all this, my childhood nickname was "Bone." (Don't ask, that's another story.) To this day, some friends from those early carefree years still call me Bone, a moniker I am hearing more often now since I'm back living in my hometown. It seems fitting somehow that, as I age, I am now experiencing Bone

Loss. Am I losing my identity along with my teeth? Likely I am, at least to the perception of society. So much of who we are deemed to be is judged by our outer appearance. This is not news. But when we begin to lose body parts or function, it's only the external changes that are noticed and commented upon. If you lose a kidney, nobody is aware of its absence unless they are told. If half your teeth are missing, everybody knows. Seeing someone on dialysis elicits a compassionate sympathetic response. Seeing a toothless crone, on the other hand, elicits only banjo music.

We will all, in some fashion or another, experience body breakdowns, whether it's from natural aging or from a premature disease process. We will all, in our own way, deal with it. As for me, I am dealing with my dental bone loss by placing the fate of my mouth in the capable, gloved hands of Dr. K. Whether I end up with an implant or a partial removable plate, a sinus hammock or a gold tooth, it will be done not in the name of vanity, but rather to help stabilize the remainder of my iffy teeth and save me from a lifetime of having to suck my meals up through a straw.

I'm hopeful this dental erosion is something that can be arrested, if not halted completely. At the very least, maybe Dr. K will be able to buy me some extra quality time with my biological teeth before introducing a boat load of foreigners into my mouth. And no doubt I'll be hearing from the rest of my body as time marches on. It might start making demands on me. I can hear it now, like a shrieking fishwife: "Quit smoking!" "Get off your ass!" "Eat calcium!" "Get a mammogram!" I'm not sure how that last one snuck in there, but I swear I've heard it before and ignored it too.

All things considered, my superior genes continue to serve me well. I can go years without getting a cold or flu and, as such, refuse to get flu shots, which I'm convinced will infect me and destroy my immune system. Anytime I get routine physicals, I amaze the doctors with my normalcy. Cholesterol, blood pressure, liver function, thyroid, Paps—normal, normal, normal. These stellar values take some of the steam out of the smug doctors' lifestyle modification speeches. Like I said earlier, I ain't gonna fix it till it's broke. I see no reason whatsoever to start squeezing myself into Lululemon and hitting the hot yoga or spinning classes until after I've recovered from my bypass operation.

When it comes right down to it, it's all a big crapshoot anyway. Professional athletes can be struck down in their prime by a sudden heart attack. People with perfect teeth can suddenly lose them. Our bodies are amazing things and will continue to surprise us with either their resiliency or their betrayals. The only thing we can count on is that with age comes change and only for the worse. You can fight it all the way to the grave in stubborn denial, or you can accept that once things start backfiring, you're starting down a slippery slope and the ride ain't gonna be pretty. Unfortunately, for better or worse, we don't all get the bodies we deserve.

In my particular case, if I keep losing bone density, I may well end up as an eighty-year-old flat sac of flesh, having to be poured into a chair where I can sit on my boneless arse, write my memoirs, and smoke and drink until . . . well, until the cows come home.

Falling from Grace

Melody Hessing

January 28. After two days of frenzied snowfall, a high-pressure system beams through the West Coast winter doldrums like a UFO, an alien presence. Vancouver winters are grey—clouds and rain, showers, drizzled days that mope along, foggy days, murky days, down-at-the-heel kind of days. I'm not a morning person. I'm still hungover from teaching last night.

But today, while I drag myself through the motions of morning tea, Tinker Bell bounces down the walls, then ricochets, spirited and bubbly, across the countertop. It's like the Hope Diamond has chandeliered the pockmarked Ikea kitchen table: Sunshine refracts on snow and carouses through the room in prisms of dancing light. It is a gem of a day, a Lazarus (I can see again, maybe I can still ski again) kind of day.

Cross-country skiing used to be one of my favourite activities. The sensation of floating through space, the slip-slide of skis on snow, the beauty of natural landscapes always enthused and replenished me. I even used to teach cross-country skiing. I've skied in the Laurentians and the Rockies, backpacked to the Egypt Lake cabin behind Lake Louise, and camped out on the Saskatchewan Glacier in February. What happened? How did I get so beaten down? Why is it so difficult to just go for a ski?

Every winter I cross-country ski on Hollyburn Mountain. But in the last few years, the drive across town to the North Shore mountains, the fuss over equipment, and the clamour of domestic chores have vetoed my efforts. Today it is clear: To prove that I'm still alive, that I haven't succumbed totally to age, and that work hasn't completely consumed me, I *have* to do this. It's only an hour there, an hour back, and after a two-hour ski, I'll feel better. Revitalized.

The machinery of preparation grinds slowly into motion. I sweep the house to find my gear: tights and wind pants and turtleneck in a duffle bag beneath the bed; gloves and toque in the hall closet. I clomp downstairs to sort through old plastic bags of rainbowed wax: black, white, special green, green, blue-green, special blue, blue, violet-blue, purple, wax for corn snow, for new snow, for old snow—old bags crazy-glued together with this stuff.

I dither around trying to figure which pair of skis to take. It is probably about zero degrees outside by now, cold for this city. My favourite old wood skis, the Birkebeiners, have a residue of purple wax on them from last winter, which will probably stick in this cold, and I don't have time to rewax the bottoms. I grab my ugly Cheapskates white plastic skis with fish-scale bottoms. Then I hunt down the bowling-shoe boots that fit the narrow three-pin bindings (the ones that barely connect you to the ski, that support grace and flexibility, but not much more). With the advent of specialty plastic boots for racing skis, telemark skis, and backcountry skis, my equipment is definitely old school. Pack, water, fleece top, parka, sunglasses, gloves, hat . . . I'm out the door!

Above the Upper Levels Highway, new snow gleams like religion. Front loaders shovel house-size clumps of snow to the side of the road. At the Hollyburn wicket, I buy my ticket, set my skis in the tracks, and begin the uphill grind, hoping to warm up in the cold.

I cruise around the bottom circuit—step, step, stutter-glide, my skis sticking in fallen hemlock needles and frozen snow. Arms and legs kick up and into the rhythm of cross-country skiing, swooping under the trees, double-poling down the crisp tracks, then crunching uphill, my breath smoky in the cold.

Over the creek, the snow is sedimented in fluffy layers, shining as if lit from within. My heart drum-rolling from effort, I herring-bone and sidestep uphill to the upper section where the snow is colder and the conditions better. From the top, the Georgia Strait stretches around the horizon; freighters loll in the harbour, and the city chunks up like a 3-D bar graph. Mount Baker Fujis the south; Mount Arrowsmith sno-cones Vancouver Island. Even the Olympics are clear. I exhale, far above the gridlock of traffic and tedium of work.

To the north, the Coast Range mountains ripple like waves in the sea. I loop uphill past snowfield lakes, on trails packed hard by track-setting machines and the bitter cold, through pillows of snow, past fairytale trees. A few pole marks dimple the snow, but nobody else is in sight.

As if I'm on a roller coaster, my skis clickety-clack down the tracks for the downhill run on the upper loop, across the main trail, and over to the steep section. I pause at the top, and then I'm flying downhill, the wind buffeting my jacket and lashing my face, my knees bent, my body hanging forward over my skis, loose, like a question mark.

Suddenly, in the midst of my descent, my skis shudder and stop as if they've hit a patch of glue. My upper body snaps forward face-first, like a ski jumper. Smack! On corrugated snow that is icy and hard and unforgiving, I cartwheel downhill in a confusion of arms and legs and skis and poles. After a sprawling pinwheel fall, I clatter to the bottom of the hill.

No bones splinter my flesh, no blood flows into the white-out snow. Shards of sunshine and freezing temperatures are the only things that register. I have been skiing for almost fifty years, and I've fallen in every possible way. But things are different this time. I feel like I've been catapulted out of my body, that I'm no longer here. I'm stunned.

A mind-body dualism is in full swing. *What's she doing? Why doesn't she get up?*

I am doing; I am trying to move.

Lying there on the snow, it's as if I have transcended myself: Part of me is outside my body, watching and observing.

I try to release my bindings by rolling onto my back, and bending my knees towards my body. My feet are miles from my hands, but I slowly make contact and snap out of my skis and bindings. Then I try to get up.

I can't.

I roll back over, facing the snow, and hunch onto my hands and knees. Then I slowly walk my hands up my poles, pulling my body up after them, until I'm in a hunched-over standing position, like a four-hundred-year-old woman with severe osteoporosis. I have no strength. I'm barely a biped.

I shuffle off the trail on the icy snow, using my poles for support. It hurts to walk, but I'm not sure how *much* it hurts. I don't know how to gauge the pain.

Someone skis downhill, picks up my skis, and sticks them in the snow at the side of the trail. Then a young woman in a red-and-blue stretch ski outfit hotshots to my side. "Can you stand like this? Can you put weight on both legs? I'm a physio, and I have experience."

"Yes, I can stand. Walking is a bit harder, though . . ."

"Well, if you can weight-bear, then you haven't broken anything.

Stretch out your legs, so they don't contract." And off she sweeps, in a hurry. I can hear her thoughts: "Pull yourself together. Just get on with it!"

But I can't walk. I can't ski down. This has never happened to me before. Problems in the past have been due to inconsequential falls and equipment failures: bindings that break, frozen toes, broken ski tips. Usually I'm skiing with other people and they help. This is something new. I'm broken. And I'm alone.

Three skiers on the ridge who witnessed my clattering descent and subsequent rusty "homo erectus" performance ski down to my side. "I think I'll need the toboggan," I manage to say, in what seems like an ordinary voice.

They nod at one another. "We'll go down to the lodge and call the ski patrol." After they leave, I hunch in my winter wonderland, watching a toy parade of skiers zip around the loop, fly down the hill, skate past me up the lip, and disappear down the other side, like Saturday at the park. I gimp over to a spot of sun, pull all my clothes from the pack and put them on. I'm shivering.

What has happened? I'm shattered but intact, conscious but fragmented. Have I been hurt or am I just stunned from the impact? How severely am I injured? And where? From my waist down to my knees, there is terrific pain if I even try to move. How could I have hurt myself so easily, when I've fallen so many times before?

It's as if I am on *the other side*. One minute I am swooping over the snow, ski-dancing, waltzing wood sticks through meadows and mountains. The next, my body is a foreign object. I watch from outside—distanced, but acutely aware that something has happened to me. My body feels familiar, but I've never hurt this intensely before. It's as if I'm a voodoo doll, strafed by needles of pain.

It doesn't compute. The weather is beautiful, the scenery spectacular. I am at the top of Hollyburn Mountain. My sense of time has melted in a frozen landscape, warped by shock, disbelief, and the sludge of inertia. In my former life—minutes, maybe hours, ago —I would have been at the car by now. But my body is here, freezing into a new time frame. I recall this sense of the turbidity of time from car accidents: The world explodes around you while you struggle to decode meaning. Nothing and everything happen all at once.

A ski machine drones over the rise in its telltale outboard stutter. The ski patrol, two young women who look like Charlie's Angels, barrels the machine over to the side of the hill, and I recognize Jenny, the park ranger from Elfin Lakes in Garibaldi Park where I backpacked last summer. As she goes through her diagnostic sequence, I explain that it hurts to walk. She presses inward at my hips. "How does that feel?"

"It's not excruciating, but it really hurts," I whimper.

"You may have a hip injury or a slight fracture, so to be on the safe side, we're going to take you down in the clamshell."

She and Patty open up the toboggan, and somehow get me into it. Tiny ripples of shivers, then big shudders of cold pulse through my body like an incoming tide. As we grumble downhill, I am Darth Vader, the embodiment of evil—and not just because of the machinery and noise of the ski machine. I have fallen from grace. I have become the injured, the poorly skilled, the inept. People stare as we go past, and I want to explain, "I know how to ski! I don't know how this happened. I'm a good skier. This could happen to anyone." But my hood covers everything but blue sky and tree bouquets, snow flowers circling the sky. We are an ice cortège, snaking solemnly downhill, a stream of cold air icicling my face. I close my eyes.

At the parking lot, it takes four people to lift me out of the clamshell casket (which has frozen shut) and onto the bed. Even with a hotpack, I am hypothermic, cold from waiting, and additionally frozen from the ride downhill. My body erupts in chills and shudders, body parts stuttering and clenched and then shivering again. It's like going into an accelerated labour in cold storage. I have no control over my body.

When the ambulance arrives, hours later, the guys shelve me into a high-tech boxy caravan of equipment as if they were packing me into the meat tray in a new fridge. They do the basic inventory—pulse, blood pressure—before we slalom down the road. I lie passively, staring up, my eyes the only things that seem to work, that I can move without pain.

It's early afternoon, but after the snowstorm, the Lion's Gate Hospital in North Vancouver is jammed. Today it should be called Heaven's Gate. Gurneys and wheelchairs hemorrhage through the door from the waiting room, packed with people so old and stiff it looks like they're already in rigor mortis. It's a northern, torpid setting of *M*A*S*H*; the enemies today are snow, healthcare cuts, and bureaucracy. Emergency itself needs triage.

My husband Jay, alerted by the ski patrol, meets me as I am shunted out of the ambulance and onto the gurney. I'm in a horizontal world, immobilized, except for my head and eyes. Whatever has happened to the rest of me has been accompanied by enough trauma that the body doesn't complain. I accept this passivity, because I am exhausted, in pain, and need help. Everyone here is just like me, bodies mummified in sheets, confined to wheelchairs or gurneys. I can't escape. There's nowhere to go.

Jay tries to penetrate the admitting desk, insinuating himself among the orderlies, ambulance drivers, and other hospital staff, to get a sense of the politics of intake. The ambulance drivers shake their heads: "It looks like a good four-hour wait until she'll be admitted. And then she has to join the queue for the X-ray."

In my mind, I'm crawling across the floor and out the door. Can you hail a cab from a crawling position? How do you get into a cab from all fours?

Jay tells them, "I've called UBC Hospital, and their Emergency isn't quite as crowded."

The ambulance guys look at one another and nod. "We can't take her over there. That's not our jurisdiction. You take her to UBC. We'll sign off."

As a parting gift, they bring me a pair of crutches. I manage to slide sideways out of bed, but the slightest move triggers jolts of immediate pain. I stick the crutches under my armpits, and then try to stand up. But I stand down. The crutches are so short that I have to bend my knees and slide my legs along the floor behind me in order to gimp forward.

"That's all we have," the ambulance guy explains. "Kids' crutches."

I drag my legs behind me like a scorpion whose curled tail has gone limp. I have to go to the bathroom. As I lower my body to the toilet, the crutches fall, and excruciating pain jolts down my legs.

Jay waits out front in his little minivan. Getting into the front seat is agony. The seat jets backward suddenly, so that I fall in, face-first, amidst the crutches. I want to drive across the border and enter a different dimension where none of this is happening. I want to get away, to go back to bed and pretend this didn't happen, to prepare tomorrow's class, to shop at the Superstore, to go home.

UBC Emergency is usually less crowded than the other hospitals. Not today. After being admitted, I stand, unable to sit down, in the waiting room. For hours.

Jay braves the Stone Angel of Admitting. "My wife can't stand any longer. Could you please bring a gurney for her?"

"You'll just have to wait your turn, sir. People here have been waiting a long time before you."

If you don't come by ambulance, you're not really sick. After an hour or so, I lurch to the concrete floor where I can lie down. Ah. Bone on concrete. Finally, someone comes out with a gurney, picks me up, and wheels me in to the emergency ward.

The X-rays are negative. I should be ecstatic, knowing that I am not seriously injured. No surgery! No days waiting in the hallway. No four-person wards with snoring and television and throngs of visitors.

But I have absolutely no faith in this process. How can this much pain be "negative"? At discharge, an orderly mutters something about "soft tissue tears." Yeah. Maybe. Abductors, adductors, hip flexors. I've heard these words in fitness class. At least I can go home! Away from discipline and control. Away from physical inertia and nowhere to lie down. Beyond institutional incompetence and an unsympathetic bureaucracy.

I'm released from hospital, dragging my legs behind me on my new adult crutches. The nurse gives me lessons about how to use them—something about heaven and hell, and which leg and crutch go first up and downstairs. I try to act like a good student, but I have a different version of heaven and hell. I have never been so happy to go home.

Today is the first day of the rest of my life. Tomorrow I won't be able to get out of bed without help. I won't be able to walk up or downstairs for weeks. The next time I walk into my classroom, it will be on crutches. In another year, I'll be scheduled for a hip replacement. This morning I was fifty-eight, *la vie devant soi.* Tonight I'm fifty-eight, over the hill.

I call in sick. I return twice to the hospital for additional X-rays. The second time, two weeks later, I get a positive reading: "fractured superior pubic ramus"—the pubic bone that connects the hips, part of the pelvic girdle. My doctor speculates that the fracture is connected to osteopenia and arthritis. I'm getting brittle.

I alternate between euphoria and pain-laced sobriety. I look at pictures of hip fractures on the web. Thank God I was not in a car accident. I do not need pins or insertions or any kind of surgery. I only need crutches.

In three weeks I'm back at work. But I can't teach on crutches. In a few more weeks, I'm back at home.

It takes a long time before I can walk, or hike, or ski again.

Two years later I'm back at Hollyburn, getting back on the horse that threw me. It's a cold grey December day, and I ski slowly back up the mountain to the site of my fall, snowplowing down the hill, looking for the exact place, but I can't be sure where it is anymore. The snow is softer, it's a grey day, the hill seems shorter. Nothing is crystal clear.

Nowadays I see mountains from the beach. The mind/body split is convenient: My body walks along Jericho Beach, looking across English Bay to Hollyburn Mountain. Somewhere up there a mountain chickadee perches on alpine hemlock, backlit by the glimmer of crystalline snow. Angels swoon on long limber wood skis and loop the loop in sexy white velcro suits, calling and falling from grace.

The Islets of Langerhans

Stephen Osborne

For most of a year my health had been deteriorating rapidly. Symptoms appeared and never went away. I presumed that I had begun to age too quickly and that I should prepare myself for death.

I was urinating every hour, and my vision was often blurry: symptoms perhaps of a collapsing prostate and advancing blindness. I hadn't been to a doctor since 1966: Was I now paying the price for too many late nights? My knees and elbows ached; I could barely pick up my feet when walking; the icy tingling in my fingers and toes I presumed to be "pinched nerves" or some form of arthritis. I began dropping things: Coins, keys, pens flew from my fingers. Most dismaying of all was the growing anger that accompanied me everywhere. This was the most disconcerting of symptoms, perhaps because anger doesn't feel like a symptom at all. I was continuously in a near-rage, and began to frighten people who had known me for years. I couldn't laugh at a joke; I couldn't make a joke. At night I could feel anger washing over me in waves. I became even angrier because I knew that there was no reason for the anger, and that made me angry too.

I was depressed and in a fog, and seemed to be constantly hungover. I couldn't sleep more than two hours at a time. I became afraid of meeting people. I couldn't bear to make an appointment. The world became heavy and there seemed to be too many things to do. I was losing weight as well, for no reason that I could see. I presumed that an unspecified "wasting disease" was overtaking me. One day in the supermarket, when I could hardly walk because my feet were hurting so badly, and my ears were ringing, a friend I hadn't seen for some time came up to me and said how well I looked (so lithe, so svelte!)—I could barely form words in my mouth. A short time after that I woke up in the morning and heard a voice say, "Osborne, you have diabetes." A simple declarative sentence.

Diabetes was merely a word to me then; I knew nothing more about it. But the directive seemed clear enough, and I went down the hill to the clinic where I learned that indeed I was suffering from a condition of the blood brought on by a defect in my pancreas, in the "islets of Langerhans," to be precise, and that the name of the disease was "diabetes," a condition described (as I would later read) by a Greek physician in 150 BC as "a melting of the flesh into urine." So it must have been my pancreas—or perhaps the islets of Langerhans—talking to me early that morning, and now I try to include my organs in my thoughts whenever I can. (An interesting exercise: Try acknowledging your spleen sometime, or your liver, or your pituitary gland.)

The doctor prescribed pills and I stopped eating sugar—for months I had been drinking root beer in cans, thinking that caffeine and sugar might get my energy up—and within a week I could feel the symptoms begin to leave my body. The fog in my head lifted, the pressure in my eyes disappeared. Slowly my body began to work as it had so long ago when I had been healthy. The tingling in my fingers went away, and I could go for half a day without emptying my bladder. I realized that I had never known what health was. Certainly I had been unable to remember it during the time of my sickness, which, as health came to me, I understood to have been about four years. Soon I was awash in normality. My eyesight improved, and I had to get out an old pair of glasses because the new ones no longer worked. I could lift things, and the house keys no longer slipped from my fingers. I began walking long distances. My bowel movements became pleasant (I hadn't even noticed how wretched they had become), and my mind became clear again, which was perhaps the greatest gift of all. I could feel myself returning to intellectual life.

The diagnosis was a gift of knowledge as well as health. Now I knew something of healing, and how ill health makes the world invisible. For a while the doctor who made my diagnosis seemed to me to be touched with genius, and it took months for the projection to wear off and for me to realize why I had stayed away from doctors for thirty-four years, for he knew almost nothing of diabetes and was unable to treat the side effects when they returned, or to regulate my fluctuating sugar levels. I had to tear myself away from him and seek out health wherever I could find it.

I turned to the "literature," a great sinkhole of medical bafflegab and self-help nonsense (a book in the public library warns diabetics not to smoke marijuana because it is "an illegal substance"), and began monitoring my own blood sugar. The pain in my legs subsided slowly, and eventually I started wearing tights under my trousers to soothe the nerve endings in my skin. Now I was walking without pain. Complications made me angry only in a mild way, because I was no longer lost in a rage. Instead I began to make my way into the world (later I discovered the therapeutic power of cinnamon and alpha-lipoic acid). I pulled on my tights in the mornings and felt like a secret Elizabethan courtier. I was learning to pick up things left undone for years, and to begin them again.

Tuning the Rig:

A Narrative of the Body

Luanne Armstrong

Pleasure comes and goes, sometimes within a single instant, but pain has real staying power.
— David B. Morris, *The Culture of Pain*

In a world where most things wind up broken or lost, our job is to tack and tune.
— Harvey Oxenhorn, *Tuning the Rig*

'm six years old, hovering on the rafters of the barn. It's spring but the back of the barn is still piled halfway up the walls with loose hay. Dust floats in the sunshine peering through the cracks in the loose boards that make a roof. A long way below, the older kids lounge, triumphant, successful.

"Jump," they yell at me. "Jump."

I hesitate. Nora, my hero, child of an alcoholic Irish dad and a kind but weary Indian mom, shrugs impatiently. Nora is three years older, has taught me to ride horses, smoke cigarettes, run away from home. For years, she was my idea of a real leader. I believed everything she told me.

"If you feel like you can do it, you can," she yells. Which makes sense. So I try it, try feeling around inside for assurance. Something in my body says, yes, go, fly, and I do. Over and over.

Farm kids. We drove tractors, hung out on tree limbs. Once I drove a pitchfork through my bare foot running to catch up with the wagon heading out to the fields. My only thought was how mad my dad would be if I got behind. I yanked it out and ran faster.

We used to race along the humped granite rocks and logs beside the lake, sure-footed as gazelles. We rode horses, climbed trees and cliffs. Crazy wild kids.

"You're just like a wild Indian," my mother would snap. And when she did, I smiled a secret happy smile.

How we live in our bodies is the part of the story of how we live in the world. The other day, I got on the bus with a book called *The Wounded Storyteller*. I read it all the way to the hospital to visit my friend Maureen, who had just had a hysterectomy. I was very excited about the book and told her about it. We talked about the book, her operation, how she felt, how she would cope on her own. Then we talked about the hospital, the nurses, laughed about the food, and I went home. On the bus, halfway home, a woman got on with a new baby, and the bus driver, who was also a woman, took the time to coo and cluck at the baby. I was envious. I wanted to coo and cluck too, but I didn't.

"He was a month early," said the woman with the baby. "I was in labour for eighteen hours for a four-pound, six-ounce baby."

"I bet it was induced," said the bus driver. "It's a lot worse when it's induced. It's a different kind of labour, see?" Everybody listened, the way they do on the bus, to this private conversation being held in public.

At the next bus stop, a woman got on with a small boy. The boy was almost bald.

"I want to go to McDonald's," she said, as though the bus were some kind of cab. The bus driver was confused.

"McDonald, there's no McDonald . . ."

"No, McDonald's, the restaurant. You have them here. We're from up north. We're staying at Easter Seal House. I've been on the bus all night and now *he* wants to eat at McDonald's." She glanced at her son, who was staring at the floor.

"Oh, okay," said the bus driver, "just hang on, I'll tell you where to go." We all watched the woman with the small boy sit down. The woman in the next seat with the baby and I smiled at each other.

When I am at the farm where my parents live, I go to church with my mother. I love our church, though I am secretly thankful that whether I'm much of a Christian doesn't seem an issue there. When I first went, I felt like a hypocrite, then ended up loving the place and the people. I feel like a kid when I'm there because I'm twenty years younger than everyone else. I sing in the choir, which is six women and me, the kid. After church, we all stay for coffee and tea, sandwiches, cake and cookies. Sometimes, on holidays, as many as twenty people attend church. That's exciting.

People exchange news about their health or their illnesses the way you would expect them to talk about a far-off war. Most people who go to our church are only a few years away from dying. They give the latest news, briefly, about their heart attacks, their cancer, their emphysema. Then they laugh. They are wonderful, these people. They laugh and they hug and they wish each other, hugely, to be as well as they can and then sail calmly back out of church to their daily lives. It's a ritual that never fails to amaze me.

My body knows more than I think it does. Once when I was young and doing many foolish things, some friends and I were drunk and stoned. We went, for no reason I will ever recall, to a park north of Vancouver, the city where I was then living. It was pitch dark. We went by a rock that was supposed to have some kind of spirit living in it, and then made our way, somehow, to the rocks and logs beside the ocean. On the way back, we began to run. Blind with booze and acid and exhilaration, I leapt from rock to rock to log to rock, each foot coming down precisely and with grace, until some more sober part of my brain realized that what I was doing was impossible and made me stop.

My parents' voices still resound in my head. "Work or starve," my dad used to say. My mother would sigh, "Time to hoist the anchor and get to work."

A good child, a good daughter, a good farmer, I have tried most of my life to follow their example. Once, years ago, I was ill with the flu. Being ill sent me into a snarling rage, sent my trying-to-be-sympathetic husband away, silent. We were homesteading then, building a log house, clearing land, working, raising four kids. There was always too much to do. We worked from morning until night, fell into bed, got up in the morning, hit the ground running, and did it all over again. We took our strength, our bodies' ability to keep up and keep going for granted. There was no time, no space for illness.

My father often spent long winter days cutting trees for firewood and burning the branches. He claimed that working around a good, big fire was a sure cure for most things. So I got up and staggered outside. I could barely walk. My head spun. I made it to the place where we had torn down an old shed and left a mess that needed cleaning.

I started a fire, dragged boards, branches, torn panelling to the fire, cursing and sweating, fighting my own weakness. The fire got taller and hotter, I sweated and fought some more. And, gradually, as the afternoon passed, the yard got clean and I got well. It works: determination, peasant stubbornness.

At least, it used to work. I tried it when I first got sick with what eventually proved to be rheumatoid arthritis. I was sore and achy and exhausted, but it was spring. The garden had to be planted, the flowerbeds weeded, the lawn mowed, the fruit trees pruned. I kept up somehow, stumbling from task to task all day, falling into bed at night.

One day I decided, as a way of curing myself, to mow the whole damned lawn—about half an acre of rocks, logs, bumps, dog bones, weeds, and some grass. I shoved the protesting ancient lawn mower around and around, sitting down often and then getting up to keep going. It was crucially important to keep going. When I finished and went inside, I could barely move. I decided a hot bath would help. (That was when I could still get into a bathtub.) It didn't. When I crawled out, I felt like my body was on fire. I was freezing and burning at the same time. I took six aspirin with codeine, wrapped a blanket around myself, sat over an electric heater, shaking, my teeth chattering. I kept fading in and out of things. Finally, I warmed up enough to go to bed. This time it wasn't working.

But it took me the last four years and finally sitting down with a friend to fill out an application for disability benefits to make me realize that this probably wasn't going away. It was time to start changing my story, the one my body had been telling me for so long, the one about being healthy, strong, and invincible.

We have a lot of mixed reactions about illness in our nice, modern, clean, technologically advanced society. We seem often to be puzzled by its persistence, its intransigence in the face of our bountiful increasing science, our vast preoccupation with safety, cleanliness, and order.

Alternative medicine talks about treating the whole person, but in my experience, and in my reading, it also reduces a person to a collection of symptoms that need to be treated, often with a lot of very expensive pills.

One day last summer, I was sitting in the yard at my son's house, drinking coffee with a young woman who is his neighbour. I probably shouldn't drink coffee, but sitting in the late August sun, becoming caffeinated and musing about stuff is one of life's great pleasures. I'm not giving it up. This young woman was serious about many things: God and self-realization and living lightly on the earth. She looked at me very sternly and asked, "Why are you still sick? What do you get out of it?"

That stopped me. But I'm quick on my feet, at least mentally. It was a serious question and deserved some thinking.

"Well," I said, after I'd thought about it for a while, "I'm not a damn farmer anymore. I can't chop wood or haul water or prune trees. I'm pretty much useless for that. So I guess I have to be a writer. Don't have much choice about it."

"You could get well if you really wanted," she said. "I have this book you should read."

I stopped her there. I've read all the books, or most of them. I know about the alternative remedies and the medical remedies. Mostly they both say, you could try this, it might work. Mostly I've tried stuff and it didn't work. I liked her first question, but what I don't need is another magic solution.

I thought about that question again, later, when I went home.

"Why are you still sick? What do you get out of it?"

I get to be lazy. I never have to move furniture again.

I get to live in the moment, feel humble, meditate, have time to think about things, read many many books. In other words, I get to have a life, just like anyone else—a life without a lot of hot baths in it, but still, enough.

Each patient brings to the practitioner a story. That story enmeshes the disease in a web of meanings that make sense only in the context of a particular life. But to understand that life and the illness experience it creates, we must relate life and illness to a cultural context. Practitioners are attracted to and repelled by both these narratives and the opportunity to interpret them in light of the patient's life world. They are attracted by the potential to understand how the person and the person's world effect and are affected by a disorder. They are repelled by the fear that the story will entangle them in confusion, which may cover over the traces of disease.

I found this passage in a book by Dr. Arthur Kleinman called *The Illness Narratives,* and suddenly, something became clear, which had felt out of kilter for me for a long time.

When I first started going to doctors, I was the one who was confused by the experience. I tried, as well as I could, to tell my story in the way I knew best, to tell the various doctors I saw how I had gotten sick, what I thought had caused it, what it had done and was doing to my life. They talked back to me in the kindliest possible way about drugs, pills, tests which had been inconclusive, using medical terms I didn't understand and had to go home and look up in the dictionary. I began to collect the peculiar things they said to me, which were so out of context that they fit nowhere in my life or my experience.

One young doctor finally said to me, at the end of a lengthy exam, "Perhaps it's just old age." Since he looked about twenty-five, and I was then forty-six, he was lucky that I was too crippled to kill him. But it was a close thing.

Another doctor looked at me and gave me some kind of truth, medically. "It's an immune system thing," she said. "We don't know much about it and we don't know how to cure it." Okay, fine, I thought, concluding rightfully enough that my story and I were mostly on our own.

As more time passed, I realized that the true story of my illness was in how I was actually experiencing it, and what was changing as a result. I realized it was held in the stories I tried to tell my friends and family, and what they heard or didn't hear. It was embodied in the stories that came back to me about how I was behaving or was expected to behave. I was deeply interested in the process of being ill, since I had never experienced it before, but I wasn't sure yet what I had learned, or how to tell it. But I knew that what I was experiencing was not a story of suffering, or self-pity, or tragedy, or even of understanding and redemption. Nor was it a metaphor for things I had experienced in the rest of my life.

But it was something that I both wanted, and needed, to pay attention to.

In *The Wounded Storyteller*, Arthur W. Frank, a professor of sociology at the University of Calgary, writes, *Sooner or later everyone is a wounded storyteller . . . . The stories that ill people tell come out of their bodies.* He describes illness as the loss of a map, or guide to identity, so that *the personal issue of telling stories is to give voice to the body, so that the changed body can once again become familiar.*

But it's not just me. Because I am now a person of a certain age, my friends are also people often dealing with illness. We exchange news of cancer, chemo, osteoporosis, drugs, herbs, naturopaths, books. The other day the same friend who was recovering from surgery said to me, "I don't know what health is anymore. I feel healthy even though, right now, I can barely move."

I am not only learning to listen to the story of my body, I am listening to other people's stories, to hear what they are really saying, to share the interest we both feel in these new, ambiguous, and interesting territories.

I am also healthy. I am a healthy crippled person who navigates the physical barriers of this life with great care. One of the subtle gifts of arthritis is that each movement needs to be carefully done, each movement carries a tiny message of pain. A careless movement or the wrong movement can be a sudden shock of pain, like brushing against an electric wire. Each movement carries its own inertia, its own heaving and sway against gravity, pushed by will and necessity. My body and I carry on a constant dialogue of limits, resistance, and necessity, a dialogue of attentiveness, of noticing.

I listen to other people's stories. I notice how people move. I watch when people climb painfully on the bus or limp after their shopping carts in the supermarket. I see more than I saw before.

The dog and I sail forth to go for a walk. He runs; I plod, tacking against gravity, hesitating between will and pain. Gravity is the major force in my life these days. I have discovered the great bliss of being horizontal, on a soft, warm, many-pillowed surface, preferably with a cup of tea and a brilliant book in hand. But if I lie there long enough, I will seize up like the Tin Man, unable to move. So I head up into the wind, lay my lumpy feet against the earth, and navigate.

The dog thinks of walks as a moral necessity. It is his fate in life to pursue walks. He is openly disapproving and disappointed if I am late with walks, or slow, or unwilling.

As we walk, various places creak, rub against one another, get stiff, turn numb. I tuck my gloved hands inside my pockets. I note each new complaint as it comes in, gauging how long I can walk, whether it's time to turn and painfully flee for home, whether I need to sit for a while on a bench at the park, watch the other dog walkers, the late evening joggers.

Until this fall, I walked on the farm. I walked carefully, lifting my feet to avoid tripping on the rough parts. I walked among the fruit trees I had pruned and picked all my life. I gave my horse away. I did less and less of the work that needed to be done.

Now I walk on pavement and the dog runs in and out of other people's yards, wild with excitement at all the new smells.

During the first year when I was really sick, I kept walking. Someone had given me this dog that I didn't really want, but he needed to be walked, so we walked. We trudged down to the beach every day, played on the sand, threw sticks. Then, every day, I would slowly and carefully climb over the rocks at the end of the beach, put my feet flat down on each rock, up the steep path where I had to stop every few feet to breathe, and then home.

I had an image of myself falling and breaking into pieces, like a badly made doll. I was afraid that if I fell, my arms and legs and bones and joints would scatter in all directions. When I walked, I picked my feet up as high as I could, which was only a few inches off the ground. When winter came, the dog and I kept walking, over the rocks that were now covered with snow and ice. Sometimes it took me several minutes to make it from one rock to the next, inching my feet along, feeling for solidity under the snow. Since I didn't want anyone to see me, we started to go at night. What I was doing was idiotic but it was also wonderful. I kept feeling my way, there in the dark, at night, in the snow, inching my way over fifteen feet of rounded beach granite, exhilarated at not falling. I was determined not to fall. It was always an adventure.

What lingers now as I walk in the city is that same sense of adventure, the sense of carefully navigating the painful yards of distance until it's time to go home and lie down in the blessed calm of being horizontal once again.

This is a new way of living in my body. When I originally got sick, I thought of pain as a cage. Now I think of it as a messenger, someone with whom I have constant, ongoing, insistent negotiation about what I can and cannot do. It is no different than the other messages the body sends—hunger, fatigue, heat, cold—except in its degree, its insistence, and its constant, present persistence.

I don't think of myself as ill. I think of myself as another kind of athlete. I use the same skills I learned from Nora, listening to know what I can do, pushing myself when I have the strength. I walk the way a marathoner runs, pushing my will against my body's strength and weakness.

I like to read. I read books of all kinds. I love travel books, and for a long while in my life I was addicted to reading books about sailing, even though I'd never been to sea nor was I likely to go. In one favourite book called *Tuning the Rig*, what stuck in my mind was the process author Harvey Oxenhorn described of tightening or loosening, adjusting all the guy wires and ropes and screws that held everything in a sailing ship together. As he puts it:

A single web distributed the tension over every inch of the rig; no part, even the stoutest mast, stood on its own; the whole thing held together thanks to counterbalanced stress, so that a change in any single part affected every other. Or, as he adds, *Regina indeed seemed like one great instrument, with her fretted shrouds, the chord of her sails, her belaying pins like tuning pegs, her hull the ocean's sounding board, her lignum vitae and mahogany, her oak and teak, her taut proud beauty and her lines that hum like harpstrings in the wind—an instrument that we, together, play.*

People who ride horses, sail boats, drive fast cars, or fly airplanes often speak of feeling these as extensions of their bodies. People who ride horses brilliantly know that such riding involves a physical communication with the horse's body, which is so sensitive and intuitive as to be almost imperceptible. The rider merely thinks of the necessary movement, and both her body and the horse's body move to accommodate that thought.

Once I had that sort of communication with my own body. Now that has changed. A distance has opened between my body and my command of it. I command it as well as inhabit it. But in this odd gap there is now some room for learning, for awareness and respect for the freedom and grace inherent in limits. Into this space has come room for rethinking my life and how I live it, room for new stories.

In *The Culture of Pain*, David Morris writes about learning to *think with pain*, a statement he calls *layered with meaning on many levels.* He adds, *This can also include assuming personal responsibility for its meaning.* Becoming ill is often a place where other people assume they have the right to explain what is happening and suggest what should be done. The function of illness for attention, for tuning into stories, is not part of the popular social discourse around illness.

Pain lives in my body as a messenger, as a secret presence hidden from others but governing my days. Nietzsche used to call his pain "dog" and take it for walks. Hemingway reportedly said, *If you've got the pain, use it.* But pain is only one small new element in the story my body has been telling me all my life. The story hasn't changed but it has been added to, enriched, altered by both loss and new knowledge, as all stories are.

Arthur Frank points out that a core social expectation of being sick is going to a doctor, and this involves what he calls, a "narrative surrender," a time when the ill person agrees to tell her story in medical terms. He calls for what he terms a "postmodern experience" of illness: *Postmodern times are when the capacity for telling one's own story is reclaimed.*

But this telling is equally dependent on the listener. Stories are a social and cultural creation, or as Frank says,

From their families and friends, from the popular culture that surrounds them, and from the stories of other ill people, storytellers have learned . . . standards of what is and is not appropriate to tell. Whenever a new story is told, these rhetorical expectations are reinforced in some way, changed in others, and pass on to affect others' stories . . . . Ill people need to tell stories in order to construct new maps and new perceptions of their relationships to the world.

I want my illness to be only a story, not a definition of who I am, how I live, or what it means. I guess I have postmodern pain, one where I get to decide what it means to me, for me. That's the very best kind.

I listen to my body tell me how far we can fly. I lay my lumpy feet against the earth, sail forth, and navigate the changing and changeable shores of this familiar land.

WORKS CITED

Frank, Arthur. *The Wounded Storyteller*. Chicago: University of Chicago Press, 1995.

Kleinman, Arthur. *The Illness Narratives: Suffering, Healing and the Human Condition*. New York: Basic Books, 1988.

Morris, David B. *The Culture of Pain*. California: University of California Press, 1991.

Anger

Dennis E. Bolen

n a cold winter some years ago, I went to Venice, ducking life. After a couple of weeks, I invited my daughter to see me. Her answer: "What's the matter, lonely over there?"

Home again, I attended the skin specialist appointment I had sought before embarking for Italy but had left too short for the doctor's three-month waiting list. As a longtime eczema sufferer, I felt half-entitled to preferential treatment, but never got it. So, better late than excessively late, here I was, six months later.

The doctor looked once around my bare body—eyes raking neck and back, legs, feet, and belly—then stopped, grim, at my chest. He pointed to a spread-out brown spot below my throat. "When did you notice this?"

"Uh. I don't think I did notice it . . ."

The thing lay at the nadir of the shirt-moulded "V," an area scorched bold by fifty years' sunlight. It was at the place where my friend Paul had warned me not to carry a pen—clasped in the folds just above the topmost-buttoned button—because of its threat as a collector of microwaves, warping the cellular structures beneath, inducing mutation, and causing trouble generally.

I had lunch with a new friend, a woman I'd been introduced to by a mutual acquaintance. She was worldly, tired, formerly ravishing. An expert at relationships, she claimed, having had so many. I instantly liked her. We yakked extensively and, of course, eventually got around to appraising our children: her two and my one. I mentioned my daughter's incuriosity. "It's worrisome. At least to me."

"Oh?"

"I mean, she's never been anywhere. I wrote her from Europe and offered her a ticket to come hang out. She scoffed at it."

"Scoffed?"

"Said something like, 'Getting lonely over there?'"

My friend stiffened. "I don't like to speculate, especially because I don't know you that well . . ."

The skin doctor peered closer at the spot. "Can you give me an idea how long it's been like this?"

"Well, it started as a mole, if I'm not mistaken. Then it sort of morphed into that spread-out brownish smear that it is right now. It hasn't been like that for long. It's not black, so I didn't give it much mind."

He drew an instrument from a drawer—a kind of scope, I could see—then flicked a switch and began scanning my chest with a coloured ray.

". . . 'Lonely'?"

"Yeah, that's what she said. In a tough-like way, too. Curt. Testy. It surprised me, I have to say. Because we've had a pretty good relationship overall, no big issues, other than my numerous marital rearrangements. She seems to have gotten used to them."

"I would say this may not be incuriosity, as you fear." My friend paused, respectful, and, I could see, hesitant. "I think she's angry."

As she spoke I received the knowledge.

"Well, I don't like it." My skin doctor is South African. It came out something like, "I doan (rhymes with 'bone') lie-kit."

"You don't, huh." I knew before I was finished speaking that my words were superfluous, routine to the doctor—the typical response of a patient on the cusp of an important receipt of information, whose mental/emotional state defaulted to an overdeveloped ability to cover any dicey situation in a blanket of words.

"Basal cell carcinoma." His pronouncement was perfectly timed to shut me up.

"What's that?"

"What you have here, I suspect." He touched my chest with his scope. The cool of the metal felt strangely reassuring.

"Anger. Yeah, that would be consistent. Her mother and I split when she was sixteen months old."

"That may not necessarily have done it."

"Maybe not, but I've been expecting retribution ever since."

"Lie back." The skin man gently guided me to prostration upon the paper-covered examination table.

"What might have caused it?"

"Many things. Heredity, injury, the sun . . ." His words trailed as action took over. With nearly alarming deftness he pulled open a drawer, thwacked on a pair of latex gloves and was flicking at a syringe. Before any more conversation could occur, the pin was in me, gently worked into the epidermis above my solar-tattooed sternum and feeding anaesthetic to the area of interest. The scalpel was brandished before I thought to expect it, glinting by the scarce light allowed by the closed slat blinds cloaking the one window of the tiny room.

"Retribution?" She put down her fork and looked at me. "Hoo-boy, you do have a back story, don't you?"

"Is it easy to see?"

"You carry it in your face. I hope you don't mind my being so blunt. It's not polite to go around telling people such things. I used to do it a lot, thought it was boldness of character and a valiant expression of uncompromised honesty." She stopped talking, then seemed discomfited by the silence. "But I don't do it so much now."

"You can tell me anything you want."

"Think you can take it?"

"I hope so. If I can't, that'll indicate something more than if I can, no?"

"Umm . . ." She wrinkled her brow. "I think that makes some kind of sense."

"Sorry to be so obscure."

"I sense I know what you were trying to say."

"I'll try to simplify. For some reason, I can take rejection from my daughter. I don't like it, but I can take it." Saying the words made me gasp slightly. I hoped it wasn't visible. "Is that a good thing?"

"Of course not."

The doctor's narrowing of eye and set of mouth transmitted all the instruction I needed: a warrant to shut my trap, while, with precision and an odd gameness—an article I'd read about surgeons' cutting obsession came briefly to mind—he carved two neat crescents into my chest. I did not watch, but the silence in the room while my skin and tissue were dissected nearly unnerved me. Then with a culinary-style flick and careful lifting of the blade, my operator finished his work and I felt instantly free.

"What do you mean, 'of course not'? Am I doing something bad by maintaining a dignified stoicism?"

She kneaded her temples with both hands. "I'm thinking, I'm thinking."

He turned away, placing instruments to the side, and returned with a thick, businesslike bandage already unfurled and ready to paste. "Leave this on for two days." He firmly set the patch where it needed to be.

I lay staring at the ceiling while the doctor washed his hands. It occurred to me that I had just had a diagnosis of cancer, short discussion of the nature of the problem, prep for an operation, the operation, post-op care, and imminent discharge. All in a matter of about ninety seconds.

"You can dress."

I sat up.

The doctor leaned against his handy bureau of medical instrument-bearing drawers, for all the world an operating room sideboard, and regarded me. "Stay out of the sun."

"I always wear a hat. I'll try to get used to that sunblock goop on my nose. I'll take vitamin D. From now on it's T-shirts instead of button-ups."

"I've forgotten for the moment, and your chart is in the other room . . ." The doctor visibly relaxed with arms folded across his chest. "Is there a history of cancer in the family?"

"Not much. Everybody dies of heart disease before anything else gets a chance at them."

"I'll send this to the lab." He gestured with his head and did not acknowledge my attempt at levity.

"Oh . . ." I pulled on my pants. "Can I see it?"

"Anger is acidic."

"That's what you've been thinking about?"

"That's what I think is important to you. Right now. Regarding this thing with your daughter."

"Anger."

"Yes."

"Hers or mine?"

She only smiled at this.

It was a coin of me, lying presentable in a petri dish. Slightly smaller than a dime. Pink-bordered.

The doctor dispassionately surveyed the sample. We both looked at it. The silence became ponderous. I required something scientific to be said.

"So what was this called?"

"Basal cell. I'm quite sure, but the lab will confirm it."

"How long will that take?"

"Usually about a fortnight."

"Oh . . ."

"Two weeks."

"Of course." I gagged slightly at the doctor's misinterpretation. I hadn't been trying to translate UK-speak: I knew how much time a fortnight was. No, I was simply taken aback at the relative eternity this part of the procedure would take in comparison to that which had preceded it.

"I'll give you a telephone call."

"Okay." I knew that here I must ask a question but struggled for content. "Uh . . . is this a serious thing?"

"Certainly."

"Basal cell . . .?"

" . . . carcinoma."

"It sure sounds serious."

"In the pantheon of cancers it is low on the scale for mortality. But if left untreated you do run a risk of metastasis." He nudged the dish with a knuckle. "This looks early. That's good."

"Glad to hear it."

"You will have a scar."

"To prove it." I smiled, but he did not.

We were both looking at the biopsy sample again.

Desperate for more instant info, I said, "Nasty little thing . . ."

The doctor turned away.

"What can I do about this?"

"Talk."

"Talk?"

"With her."

"I guessed that. Seriously, too, I guess. It'll take some considering,

I don't want to blow it. I may only get one chance. I suppose I should be prudent? Diplomatic?"

"What's your daughter like? Does she have trouble with full-on confrontation?"

"Hmm . . . Yeah."

"Oh."

"She's . . ." I had to calculate. "Twenty-two. But she still uses the old hands-over-the-ears, I'm-not-listening childhood trick whenever I want to discuss something heavy. It's like a private joke between us."

"So you joke around."

"Sure. It's the best part of our relationship."

"Well then, at least there's hope."

"You could say that about anything, though."

"I suppose . . ."

Things went slack then, over the coffee.

She picked at her dessert and looked up. "Was it true?"

I managed enough concentration to process back to what she was most likely referring to. Though I located it in an instant, an unexpected trouble blocked my vocal passages. It took some effort to continue on my candid way. "Yes." I set my eyes into hers. "I was lonely." I looked away. "Of course I was."

"Oh . . . I'm . . ."

" . . . sorry you asked."

We made small talk in the dying seconds of lunch.

Striding from the clinic, the dressing hidden under my shirt so nobody could see what I'd been through, I felt only a slight chafe but didn't feel especially well. There was jelly at my centre: something loosened and shifting in a tender place. I put it down to shock—having so abruptly required the ruthless skill of a grave professional. Too, there was a benign guilt. After all, I'd just undergone a cancer operation, had had no pain, and walked now in the confidence of an excellent prognosis.

I wondered if people could see anything in my face.

How to Survive the System: Tips for Boomers

J. Cates

I was grocery shopping in a Superstore when I took, as a friend put it, a nosedive into the frozen peas. It's okay for her to talk to me like that—we're members of the same club. She paid for her membership with a bilateral mastectomy; I bought mine with a cardiac arrest. After her operation, we tried to think of ways she could tell any new boyfriends that she was, shall we say, a couple of prows short of a *Queen Mary*. I suggested tasteful euphemisms like "hooterectomy" and "disemboobment," but she didn't care for them.

But anyway. We're all destined to become members of the club—some of us are just more involved in it than others are.

I want to give a few tips to the boomers who are beginning to crash upon the medical profession like waves on rocks. Some of us almost-sixties got a head start with our hearts and hooters and strokes and such, so why not share and tell our pals what they'll be dealing with? And who.

First, though, I was just goofin' about the nosedive into the frozen peas. I have no memory of it. I could just as easily have done a header into the halvah or a leap into the lemons. I remember putting a couple of packages of noodles into my shopping basket, and the next thing I knew I was sitting in a hospital bed three days later, talking to my sister. She said I'd been more or less coherent the whole time, but a heart incident can wipe the short-term memory, and I don't remember a thing about those three nasty days—and good, because who needs to know what all went on?

She said I argued with the doctor in the emergency ward. He wouldn't let me go home. Words were exchanged. I flipped him the bird. Then they flew me to a big-city hospital with a big-city cardiology department. Later, I was pleased I'd had the presence of mind to flash the finger in spite of my condition. I was annoying to officialdom even while hooked up to machines and mother-nekkid. Damn, I'm good.

Here's them tips. Mainly, don't be overly respectful of anyone. Waking up a medical prisoner tends to generate a bit of the old Stockholm Syndrome, but don't give in to it. If you do, they win.

Medical people are working stiffs like any other and will sometimes screw up. If this is bothersome it's not because they fail to be perfect, but because we *expect* them to be perfect.

Some of them may be caring, selfless humanitarians, but let's not dwell on them. Screwups are more interesting to us. We're funny that way.

The first people you'll see when you wake up in a hospital are probably going to be nurses, and, sad to learn, they're about the same as any kind of staff in any kind of job, even the human meat-processing industry. A few nurses will be excellent; most will be competent but nothing special; and a few of them you wouldn't want taking care of a dog, much less a person. Your period of being in awe of nurses will expire at about the time one of them accidentally yanks out your intravenous line because she's not paying attention, maybe still thinking about last night's episode of *ER*, wondering why her own life pales in comparison and where it all went so terribly wrong.

The intensive care ward, after serious surgery, is a sub-habitat with its own peculiarities. After you wake up, see if you can spot the nurse who'd be most likely to sneak you a mickey of rum and a deck of smokes. She won't, but she might boost your morphine a tad. And we had great fun when she yanked out my catheter for me. Oh, how we laughed. Guys, you might want to be ready for that, so you can explain that some things change in size in certain situations, and it's bound to be smaller when you're sick, but at other times will be a lot bigger, honest. Try a Pinocchio analogy.

Intensive care is not without its good times. When one of the nurses said, "Hey, this guy's oxygen ran out; he's been breathing room air for the last hour," we all enjoyed a hearty chuckle.

Don't respect doctors too much either. Your supply of doctor-worship will run low when they keep calling you by the wrong name. I mean, the cat's vet can remember my name, but a cardiologist can't?

I found out one pretty cool thing about doctors: Even if you flip 'em the bird, they still have to take care of you. Check it out for yourself. Isn't that great? Try it with a civilian, see what it gets you. (I must mention that some months later I had an appointment to see the doctor I'd flipped off, and he kept me waiting in his office for forty-five minutes. So, even though they may have trouble with their patients' names, in other ways, they have *very* long memories.)

You won't be having a lot of discussion with doctors anyway. If a patient asks a specific question, they'll answer it, but if a patient doesn't know what questions to ask, the doctor won't volunteer much. Giving patients more information than they ask for might confuse the poor things. I swear, I want to make a card for patients who are exhausted and full of strange drugs, so they can just hand it to their doctors. It will read as follows: "Please give me all the information I'd ask for if I knew the right questions to ask and if I wasn't exhausted and full of drugs, and if we both didn't know there was somewhere else you'd rather be."

That's why you gotta display the digit to a doctor now and then—otherwise they can become uppity and start feeling too God-like, and then they won't tell you damn-all. God doesn't have to explain anything.

One thing every over-fifty has learned is that the world is full of pipsqueaks, and every younger person should be considered a pipsqueak until proven otherwise, and being a doctor or nurse doesn't mean they're not also pipsqueaks. So don't let them push you around.

The practice of medicine isn't entirely about what the patient wants, but also what course of action is the least likely to result in one of those pesky lawsuits. This is why we have the word "overcautious" in the dictionary, somewhere between "overbearing" and "oversimplify." It might be used in a sentence, thus: "Even if a doctor thinks a treatment can be overcautious, his lawyer won't." Or: "Doctors would rather be called 'overcautious' than 'defendant.'" (An interesting little prefix, "over." It combines nicely with such words as "zealous" and "medicated," but see how awkward it sounds if you try to combine it with words like "helpful" and "informative.")

Many of the things they'll do to you in a hospital come under the heading of what doctors call "defensive medicine." Understand that, and you understand modern medical technique.

There's one group I can't find fault with: the surgeons. I mean, imagine having a complete stranger carve you open like a fresh-caught trout and stick his hands into your chest cavity—isn't that just too weird and icky?—and then you're able to go home a few days later with only a handful of Tylenol.

Of course, what do I know, really? I was asleep. Maybe my surgeon smoked while he worked and dropped ashes into me and rinsed me out with the dregs from his coffee cup. I mean, how would I know? But I choose to think surgeons are great, because you can't fuss over every little damn thing.

You won't see much of the hospital's rank and file, who scurry in darkness below the ground. Technicians will ascend now and then to take blood and stick things into you. My ministering angel whined on and on and bloody on about how much she hated her job the whole time she was using me for poking practice.

My suggestion? Berate the twenty-somethings from the get-go—better to have them live in fear than encourage them to be condescending. Almost the first thing boomers will notice in the hospital is the unlimited capacity for condescension displayed by the young. Crush them like roaches. Break their spirit. They can't hit back.

Then there are the kitchen people. They worship cream of wheat because it doesn't clog the toilets when all that white crap gets flushed. They use cream of wheat for currency, there, in the dark, where they fear for their lives should they show their faces in the light of day. And rightly so.

Don't think life turns into a bowl of cherries if you survive the hospital to see the light of day again. After you flee the place, you still have to deal with doctors, labs, and clinics on the outside.

Their staff are invariably short, blonde, slightly overweight girls of twenty-something who are only too willing to send you chasing all over the province for tests you could have had done practically next door to your home. It's just easier for them to send you chasing all over the province than to make a few phone calls, while they ponder the last episode of *Grey's Anatomy*, wondering why their own lives are so lacking in romance and where did it all go so terribly wrong.

Don't believe anything these bimbettes tell you. *They are not on your side.* For that matter, no one in a hospital is completely on your side, except maybe the other patients, and they can be incredibly sweet because they're in our club. Medical people are in a different club, and will choose whatever treatment they want to, or whatever they think you want, or whatever they think you *should* want. What they won't do is ask what you *do* want. If you're lucky, their agenda will coincide with yours. Just remember: An educated guess is still a guess.

So think kind thoughts about Tommy Douglas and enjoy the drugs. The aging hippies among us will appreciate the wisdom of that advice. As the free pharmaceuticals drip into you, see if you can still say "far out" as if you really mean it. Your attending pipsqueaks can't understand how much more expensive dope has become since the sixties. Lawsy, child, the prices nowadays.

As for me, three years later, I'm pretty much back to normal and back at home. I have a new apartment; it's between a hospital and a graveyard, and I think that's great. And my friend sans rack is still dating.

Maybe all of this will help when you're an active member of the club and getting ready to move on. Eventually there won't be anyone left in the club—only echoes of us all, and those won't last long.

One day, in my hospital room, a four-bedder in cardiac central, an old man of maybe eighty was talking to his doctor, and I pulled a curtain around my bed to give them privacy, but I could still hear them talking.

Doctor: "The tests show one of your carotid arteries is completely blocked, and the other one's too far gone to be helped."

Old man: "Well. That's it then."

Doctor: "Is there someone who can pick you up?

Old man: "My son's coming to get me."

Clever of him to escape the clutches of the hordes hell-bent on keeping his body warm and moving for as long as they could.

When the old man left a few minutes later, he looked around the edge of my curtain and smiled and waved goodbye to me. He seemed content and was very pleasant. Graduating from the club. Going, as they say, in style. Smile and wave goodbye to us, old partner. We'll meet again in a better place than this, speed the day.

Body Clay

Ruth Murdoch

Years ago, I made a bowl out of clay. I wrote: "The clay, a sacrament; its essence, prayer. My hands shaping it with water: benediction, baptism. My fingers finding its shape, the way it is suddenly necessary to find the softest place between holding and not holding, and rest there. This bowl holds mountains, rivers, raging currents, the ways they move and shape each other. It holds everything, and holds nothing back." In clay I keep movement alive and remember possibility; in clay I dance. Clay brings me to my body: sensuous, in pain, frozen, and full of beauty. Clay embraces all of me and is my mirror. For a while, I forgot this.

In my art therapy office, bags of old hard clay accumulate—clay too hard to shape, too hard to do anything with except start over. For months, I assumed I would discard it, but for some reason, I didn't. Even the bag on the art table is growing hard; nobody has used it for months. I've noticed this, but it has taken me a long time to act. Last fall, I carried boxes of my sculptures out into my garden, where they over-wintered and turned back into the earth. Almost one year later, I bring the hard clay home. I carry the bags downstairs and fill two buckets: one with grey clay and one with red. The task: reconstitution. I will find a way to work with the unworkable. I add water and wait.

HISTORY

I was born in 1959, one month premature, and with a life-threatening abnormality in my heart: a double aortic arch, which constricted my esophagus and trachea. I spent the first two months of my life in an incubator. I had corrective heart surgery at seven months, but because of infections and other complications, the doctor told my parents for a year that I was dying. Another doctor told them I would be "a little vegetable." I can't imagine what that must have been like for them. I know my arrival threw my family into chaos. I still remember the day I was told my heart was functioning normally. I was eight years old, and I had learned that my most important task in life was to survive.

I was also born with one hand; my right arm ends just below my elbow. The doctor reacted by quickly removing me from the birthing room. His words: *Mrs. Murdoch, you have a daughter, but . . . well . . . she's not perfect.* He took me from my mother, not because of my serious congenital heart condition, but because he thought she needed protection from the shock of my apparent imperfection. Even though this wasn't true and she demanded to see her daughter, even though I was a newborn baby and I couldn't have known what was going on—somehow I learned this: the idea that people might need protecting from the truth of who I am. At three years old, when someone remarked on my missing hand, I proudly announced, "That's a hand, another kind of hand!" My arm is at my foundation, shaping my identity, my personality, how I am in the world. I have always felt different, and my arm has been the most visible manifestation of that difference. It has never held me back, but rather has repeatedly brought me closer to my strengths and abilities. It sparked in me the fierce independence and determination that propel me forward.

At seventeen, I had back surgery to correct scoliosis. A steel rod was implanted to stabilize the curvature, and my back was fused. At twenty-nine, when I started to experience back pain, I consulted with an orthopaedic surgeon, who told me that my spine was degenerating. I learned that my pain is a result of the surgical techniques used in the day, and that most scoliosis patients who had their surgery in the 1970s are experiencing this. My back is relatively inflexible and cannot absorb shock the way normal backs do. Consequently, the regions below and above the rod experience elevated levels of stress. The orthopaedic surgeon's words painted a bleak picture: degeneration, increasing pain, progressive disability. He said that when the pain became unbearable, the only recourse would be more fusion, which would, in effect, shift the point of impact into my sacral region. The solution would inevitably become a part of the problem. His words: *By the time you are forty, you will be in so much pain that it will be unbearable.* With my breath, I drew his words in like magnets to old beliefs. They circulated; they bounced off my arterial walls. They flowed in my bloodstream and got into everything. And then they hardened. When I turned forty, I turned to him and spoke to the air, "You were wrong. I am in pain, but you were wrong. It is not unbearable." However, I knew that the degeneration was progressive, that my pain would increase, and that I would be disabled. This knowledge was in my body, and I stooped with the weight of it.

Also at twenty-nine, I convinced my doctor that the irregularity of my menstrual cycle was beyond the range of normal. She referred me to an endocrinologist in Vancouver. Following the requisite blood tests, I learned I was experiencing premature menopause. After eliminating all other possible reasons for this, he concluded that repeated X-rays of my lower back had likely damaged my ovaries. Apparently, radiation from X-rays gathers in our bodies, and its effects are cumulative.

I was learning firsthand how decisions about medical procedures and treatments are made. There are no absolutes. There is never a perfect treatment, pill, surgery, or procedure. Medical decisions are the result of weighing benefits and risks. Each X-ray I had was justified because the doctor considered his need to see into my body greater than the dangers of the radiation. This is what I see: Each of the three orthopaedic surgeons I consulted over the years made his decision in isolation. No one looked at the bigger picture. No one asked me how many times my lower back had been X-rayed. Never was I told of the possible consequences.

That year, my orthopaedic surgeon recommended that I continue having annual X-rays of my spine. My endocrinologist recommended that I start taking hormone replacement therapy. I felt caught in a frightening trap—no matter what I chose, the risks felt too great. The best way to avoid further iatrogenesis was to stop accepting what doctors offered me. I said no to both.

REFLECTION

In the house where I grew up, the green upstairs bathroom had a wall of cupboards above the counter, which extended the entire length of the room. Two of the doors on these cupboards were mirrors, and when you opened them, the mirrors faced each other, creating infinite reflections in both directions. I remember standing in-between the two mirrors, turning around and around, looking at myself reflecting back and back and back. This memory is among my roots, deep in the beautiful ground I am growing in. It has become a metaphor that still lives inside me. As an adult, I see this same kind of resonance all around me. From a point of origin, the impacts (and images) may reverberate forever. That's how it is in my forty-seven-year-old body. Think about how sounds can reverberate in the air. We hear the sound, and then we hear in its waning a growing distance, as if the sound is travelling away. It's like that, but what I hear moves towards me. The words wind their way into my core, the sound growing more muffled on the journey in. For years at my core there has been silence, stiffness, and the suspension of movement.

MOVEMENT

So when my physiotherapist says, *Everything's collapsing*, it isn't something that I can just hear and then pass off or let go. That phrase comes in, and I, like an auger, grab it, hold onto it, and work it in. His words have stung me, but this professional man is a good person: compassionate and proficient at what he does. When he tells me that everything's collapsing, he imagines he's explaining something. For example, why I have been in such pain, why my pelvis goes out of alignment with the slightest movement, why I can't do what I used to do. He doesn't see what I see. The image: a tangled heap of bones, tissue, muscle, and organs. A collapsing, mangled mess of whatever it is that is the flesh of who I am. I am afraid that I can't put myself back together . . . I can't do this anymore. I can't. "Push," he says, "push against me as hard as you can. Push . . . PUSH . . ," At his prompting, everything in me goes into pushing my pieces back into place, over and over and over. I push against my fears—

that degeneration is inevitable, that I don't have enough strength left. That I am disintegrating.

I learn that my muscles have adapted to the misalignment and have forgotten what is normal. Now, each time we push my pelvis into place, my body reacts with a deadweight pain. I drive fast, trying to get home before the pain descends. I take painkillers and lie down, afraid to move. After each adjustment, I go into battle as my muscles try to pull my pelvis back out of alignment, and I fight against that pull. He tells me that the first forty-eight hours following realignment are critical. For weeks, this is happening every three or four days.

My physiotherapist is trying to tell me that there is a way to fix this, that my body isn't what it seems. Or that at least there is a way to do the best I can with what I have. He doesn't know that, by now, it's hard for me to hear this, and his words are becoming lost. Or: I have stopped listening because pieces of my body have hardened, aren't where they are supposed to be, where they used to be, where I can find them. Or: I am lost and this is the place I remember: where my body is what it is and works against me, where the despair in my bones knows there is nothing I can do, where my body is hard clay.

I hold myself stiff as a board. I must take tiny steps only. I must move my entire body together—no twisting. My pelvis, torso, and head must always point in the same direction as my feet. My knees must never be more than one foot apart. No walking on uneven ground. No running. No jumping. No snowshoeing. No dancing. No digging. No squatting. No gardening. The seasons become identified by the things I cannot do. I picture myself coming loose, trying to salvage the pieces, trying to find places for everything inside me. Where do I fit this despair? Where do I fit this fear? Where do I fit this determination? What is happening inside me? I should know the extent of the degeneration. I should be X-rayed. I haven't been X-rayed for eighteen years. I begin weighing my fear of knowing against my fear of not knowing, and they are in perfect balance. From the middle of this fear, I request X-rays of my entire spine—from the base of my skull to my tailbone. The X-ray technician is hard. She tells me to stand here and move my body there. When I don't follow her instructions, she jerks and twists me in ways my physiotherapist says are forbidden. I am afraid that my pelvis will go out again.

I am in my physiotherapist's office when he receives the radiology report by fax. He reads it aloud. We learn that the degeneration is still focussed in my lower lumbar spine. There is no degeneration in my upper back; in fact, the degeneration has not spread much in eighteen years. I ask questions, trying to grasp the meaning of the report. Why then has my pain felt so much worse? Why do I suffer crippling muscle spasms in my upper back? Why do I feel so much more disabled than I did at twenty-nine? He tells me that my posture is the problem, and that I must start standing straight. All these years, I didn't know I hunch forward as I walk. Or, I believed that bent is just the way I am. The orthopaedic surgeon predicted progressive disability, and I simply believed him without question. Year after year, there was abundant and increasing evidence that he was right. My body does not move that way; my body is hardening; my body hurts—all these years, my body is what it is and works against me.

Now this report is telling me that he was wrong. I am learning firsthand about the power my beliefs have to shape my experience. My physiotherapist tells me that my body is capable of good posture. I resolve to stand up straight, forcing my body to stand and move in ways it has forgotten. Although my stiff movements are full of pain, my awareness increases. I begin to notice a relationship between pain and posture, to understand how, over the years, my body has made my pain visible. It becomes a discipline of will, consistent practice, and mindfulness that will colour my days for months to come. He talks about developing core strength, and tells me if I develop these deep muscles, they will hold me together. He tells me I can heal, that I can grow less disabled than I have been for years. He refers me to a personal trainer.

When I start to see the personal trainer, my pelvis still goes out of alignment all the time; I am still in a lot of pain. At the first appointment, I lie on a mat on her office floor, and she teaches me how to get up safely. She shows me how to find my core muscles, how to isolate them, and how to work them. She uses a tool to gauge the level that my core muscles are contracting. I am learning words like "activate." She shows me images of core muscles so I can see their massiveness and can understand their capacity to protect me. After just three weeks of training, my pelvis stays in alignment for one month. I arrive at her door week after week, my face hard with pain and determination. She too challenges my beliefs about my body, challenges me to rethink my relationship to what is happening. I say to her, "I don't think my body moves that way."

She responds, "Well, Ruth, I think that it does."

Slowly, I am deconstructing old beliefs and making room for new ways of being in this world. As my capacity to work my muscles increases, she advances my exercises, and I begin to feel the strength growing inside me, to think of my body as malleable, to imagine the doctor's oppressive words dissolving.

I am sitting with my buckets of softened clay. I pour the water off the top and spread the mucky, settled mass on a sheet of plywood. As the excess moisture evaporates, I begin to gather up the clay and work it. It sticks to my hands and is a mess at first. However, with time, and as I work it, the clay slowly gains body in my hands, and begins to hold its shape. I begin to wonder what I am creating. I see movement in what has been frozen, rigid, and still. The Taoists would tell me that a finished image lies in the clay, waiting to be uncovered. My task is ultimately a simple one: to feel the image in my being and allow it to emerge. This, above all else, is an act of faith. The clay will embrace all of me and is my mirror. I remember.

No Death

Doreen Colmer

People like me. I am fun to be around and capable of fitting in socially to most situations. I know what makes good cocktail party conversation and I know what doesn't. Cancer, for example, is something to avoid when trying to keep things light.

It's been four years since my diagnosis, and the fact that I have stage four breast cancer rarely comes up anymore. I think it's because people don't associate me with the disease. It does not define me; how I've handled it does.

Stage four breast cancer is about as bad as it gets. There are other terms for my disease: "advanced cancer," "metastasized cancer," "late stage," "end stage." I prefer to keep it simple. I call it "the bad kind." I have long since outlived the statistics, which are bleak at best. In a nutshell, I was a goner.

The few who do survive are said to have gone into spontaneous remission, which is another word for "we have no way of explaining this." My remission has been anything but spontaneous. It has been well planned and anticipated.

When people ask me how I'm feeling, I'm always positive. People don't treat me like I'm dying because I'm not dying. I'm not even sick. When people see how healthy and vibrant I am, it becomes easy to believe what I've been telling them all along: I will beat it.

I have no physical symptoms of cancer. Other than a couple of days of post-op recovery, I have been perfectly healthy. Other than having breast cancer spread to both lungs and almost every bone in my body, I'm not the least bit uncomfortable. What makes me uncomfortable—*very* uncomfortable—is the thought of having cancer. The thought of dying from it is unbearable.

The only thing that gives me comfort is the belief that I can and *will* defy the odds. Anything else is just bullshit.

Someone once tried to console me by talking about how exciting heaven would be. She made it seem as if I were privileged in some way, and actually implied that the afterlife was somehow better than the life I had at home, with my husband and two young sons. She even asked if I was at all anxious to meet God. Um . . . No, I'm not. I figure if God and I are meant to be together eternally, then what's the big rush? I was thirty-eight at the time, not eighty-three.

Many people have used talk of an afterlife as a way to comfort me. "There is no death," they say. "Death is not to be feared," they say, "because there is no death."

At first I just went along because I wanted to make them feel better. I agreed, nodding, wiping tears away. *Certainly, eternal life, definitely, there is no death, absolutely, I hear you.* Now I speak up. I tell it like it is.

My spiritual self may not die, it may live on—fine, whatever—but there is no doubt that this five-foot-seven, one-hundred-and-mumble-mumble-pound body will, in fact, die.

If this disease is the end of me, my death will be very real.

How many times will my boys have to say their mother is dead? Probably hundreds On dates, they'll be asked about their mother, and they'll have to say I am dead. They'll be like all those kids in the family movies. Somebody's parent is always dead, the kid's life is ruined, and then something happens in that kid's life to make him whole again. It usually involves a pet or some friendly sea creature. Believe me, I've seen them all.

If I die from this disease, my kids will be at all the walks for breast cancer. It will become our family's cause. They may even wear T-shirts with my picture on it—in loving memory of their dead mom.

I wonder how many times my husband will have to say his wife passed away. If he is fortunate enough to find love again, I will become the "first wife," and to my children, I will be the "real mom."

"My first wife died from breast cancer," my husband will say. "My real mom died when I was young," my boys will say.

For as many people who have denied the existence of death, there are even more who think they'll be hit by a bus. They say it so casually, as if it were likely.

When I was told my cancer had spread, my oncologist put her hand on my knee and said, "I know this is bad, and I am so sorry; I know you feel awful, but we are all going to die. I could get hit by a bus tomorrow." She actually said that: *I could get hit by a bus tomorrow.*

What is it with buses—do they really hit that many people?

Other well-intentioned people have also said that to me. That "hit by a bus" metaphor has been used many times by people who are genuinely trying to make me feel better.

At first I would wipe my tears and agree, just so they would feel like they had given me comfort. *Yes, I hear you, die tomorrow, uh-huh, hit by a bus, I know.* Now I gracefully tell them the difference between their bus and mine. They need to know this.

I remind them that if they are afraid of being hit by a bus, they have the option of never leaving the house. I don't have that luxury. I've got some crazy out-of-control bus following me wherever I go—the kind of bus in a horror film, driven by some freak who's hell-bent on taking me out.

And, unlike most bus victims, I will not be so lucky as to die instantly. My bus driver is a sadist who will slow down to run over me, inch by inch. My family and friends will have to stand by and watch helplessly while I get run over by the big ugly bus, knowing that when it is finished with me, I will be dead.

Hopefully, one day there will be an end to buses hitting people, and that saying will become a thing of the past. In the meantime, I'll work with it. I'll give it a little tweak and make it my own.

My bus driver is on strike.

This bus is no longer in service.

Thanks for the brake.

Tied with Black Grosgrain Ribbon:

Letters to the Insurance Adjuster

Crystal Hurdle

October 21

Dear Insurance Adjuster:

Thank you for getting in touch with me via voicemail. I'm not a little alarmed to note that you sound approximately twelve years old. Is it a disguise, or are you a wee boy? Far be it from me to be accused of ageism, but my disability is of some consequence, so is it possible my case file could be allocated to a grown-up?

Sincerely yours,
Case File 717185

October 22

Dear Insurance Adjuster:

Thank you for letting me know that my disability claim has been accepted until October 24. Judging by the date, this is a trick or perhaps a test. Do not fear—I am up for the challenge! I will do my best to fit the estimated six weeks of recovery time into two days.

Sincerely yours,
Case File 717185

October 25

Dear Insurance Adjuster:

Thank you for the new form #73 that you requested me to fax you from my bed where I am presently marooned. I understand that you are delighted by the seeming ease of the tick-box system.

So it comes to this: no sabre, no sword, just a pen. Perhaps the pen really is mightier than the sword. How can you be an enemy with such antiseptic requests? Or perhaps you are trying to trick me. Aha! I am up, but barely, for the challenge.

I have duly placed ticks in the corresponding boxes for "patient can incline head at a forty five-degree angle," "patient is capable of manipulating two or more fingers on one or more hands," and "patient is to some degree ambulatory."

How this translates into "patient is her usual lively, curious, energetic self, ready to leap around the classroom and to write report-like comments on student essays, during repeated ten- to twelve-hour work days," I am not exactly sure. I expect another test will follow forthwith. My pen is at the ready! Perhaps your sending form #74 will provide an answer to this perplexity.

Sincerely yours,
Case File 717185

P.S. Having no fax machine in my bedroom, I will seal form #73 into an envelope and have my husband post it. My present ambulatory skills do not allow for the two blocks to the mailbox.

October 30

Dear Insurance Adjuster:

Thank you for your visit earlier today, during which time you tracked mud over the threshold onto my clean floors. No invitation had been extended, but you do have certain rights, I understand. I am learning. You seemed exuberant to see a freshly polished dining room table, a clean carpet, and seasonal decorations.

These niceties have been hard won. I dust a room a day for exercise, with frequent rests in-between. I make sure my husband keeps the carpet clean because I find myself frequently napping on it.

Over the last three weeks, on occasional trips to the basement, I have retrieved one decoration at a time. Now, I expect the decorations to be up for the next few months, as I haven't the energy to put them away, never mind to set out more for a new holiday. In any case, the witches and bats, dark souls, seem fitting for my season. My imaginative vision sees death, not birth. Death to germs, death to unsanitary conditions, breeding grounds. The filth on your muddy boots.

Because I am well enough to clean does not mean that I am well enough to work unless you can obtain for me part-part-part-part-part-time custodial services at the college.

Sincerely yours,
Case File 717185

November 5

Dear Insurance Adjuster:

No, yes, I am without diagnosis still, yet.

Thank you for checking up on me. It's nice to feel needed. I hope you will recommend my fashion statement to all other clients under your care: dirty sweats, unwashed hair, and an ice pack wrapped in a tea towel on the head. It was clearly a mistake to have left my door ajar, the sill glistening from Lysol. My body is my house.

You understand that, as much as I would have liked to invite you in for tea, I simply could not. Yours, after all, was hardly a social visit.

Sincerely yours,
Case File 717185

November 8

Dear Insurance Adjuster:

Thank you for pointing out the egregiousness of my doctor's claim that I am sick. Sotto voce, you note that some doctors are more than generous, allowing five years for cancer, two months for, say, a cold. While I appreciate your desire to have a rapport with me, I hope you won't mind if I suggest that it would be better all around were you to go to bed early, eat all your greens, and listen to your elders, including wise doctors, particularly my doctor.

Sincerely yours,
Case File 717185

November 10

Dear Insurance Adjuster:

Thank you for advising me that further disability payments will cease without corresponding paperwork from my doctor. What, pray, do you wish, as my file folder must be a foot high with results of scans, biopsies, treatments tried? My doctor is as sick of this as I am.

Perhaps a photocopy of the planetary outcropping on my infected leg, should I be able to drape it over the Xerox machine? Or a note from me suggesting that my doctor is not sick? She is despairing, she is weary, she is stumped, but she is not ill. Perhaps an origami snowflake to add beauty to your hard, hard life?

Perhaps a co-authored poem about return to health being less than linear, as is your thinking? Or perhaps some soggy tissues made into clumps of statuary from our tears?

Sincerely yours,
Case File 717185

November 14

Dear Insurance Adjuster:

Thank you for suggesting that an immediate return to work will speed my recovery. I am too weary to fight you. I'm guessing you are the enemy. There has to be one. Your wish is my command.

I will plan mini-lectures of not more than five minutes to allow for the results of nausea and diarrhea. I can surely read the thermometer as I circulate to check students' work, provided that my tottery legs will hold me erect.

As my classes are of four hours' duration and I've not been awake for more than three hours in a row, I'll do my best to find pertinent filmstrips to show during the last hour. Have you, in your wisdom, any suggestions for worthy titles?

Or perhaps, given the stresses of college life, students will enjoy napping along with me. We will dream deeply of a parallel universe in which evil is vanquished, and Health reigns supreme.

Sincerely yours,
Case File 717185

P.S. I'll need your advice on how to keep the ice pack at a suitable cryogenically appropriate temperature.

December 1

Dear Insurance Adjuster:

Thank you for wondering what I am doing at a health spa while you play Mr. Scrooge, cutting me thinner and thinner disability cheques.

The masseur is pummelling out the old pain with new; the baptismal sulphur water is making all my skin as purple as the infected patch.

Trust me that this is therapy, not pleasure. Trust me that this place is as much a workhouse as yours. Trust me that I am struggling to get better, to speed up my recovery, so that your cheques can thin to nothingness, just as you would wish during this festive time, when all good little boys get what they ask for.

(I see that's what you are, all you are: a good little boy, nothing to have feared.)

Sincerely yours,
Case File 717185

P.S. Please find a new pair of fingerless gloves, size extra small, under separate cover. The best of the season to you and yours.

Finding an Ending

Janis Harper

'm not sure if I died on the operating table. It's been almost three years since I had my colon removed, three years of normal-seeming life. But how do I know this isn't a transition phase from death to whatever comes next—that for me it seems like three years, but that's just how I perceive time, which I already know is illusory. Maybe I need this "time" to experience it all some more, to say goodbye, to love the people in my life more, to do what I think needs to be done before I can tear myself away.

Part of me waits for the tear in the fabric to appear, without warning, suddenly: while I'm gazing into the sweet face of my twelve-year-old son as he's telling me about his day at school; as I'm walking through the familiar tree-lined streets in my neighbourhood; when I wake up to pee at four in the morning. It will happen when I'm most comfortable, content, fully in the present, pow! A crash of unfamiliar noises, surgical instruments, blinding light of the operating room, my surgeon talking in urgent tones to the nurses, erratic beeping of the heart monitor: "We're losing her!" Then, gradually, the visuals will come in. I'll see a flurry of activity in the OR from above, someplace around the ceiling. The heads of my surgeon and the nurses, myself lying flat on my back, two-dimensional, covered in a white sheet. Why am I seeing this when I was just having a breakfast of Honey Nut Cheerios with my son? Then I'll know it's true—what I've always suspected since

I woke up in a groggy stupor with a stapled stomach and tubes stuck in everywhere. I really did die.

Beginnings are the hardest, writing teachers like to say that. Once you get going, the rest falls into place. I disagree. Beginnings are easy. I've always known where and how to start. Endings seem like they should be easy, too. Closure—one gets it one way or another, either consciously at the time or in reflection after the fact. These are harder to pinpoint, though. I think, with endings, you just have to make them up. They're more arbitrary, more ambiguous. When you're born, there you are, suddenly, where you weren't before. When you die . . . well, that's what this is all about, isn't it. I'm not sure how this story will end either, but I'll just have to have faith that I will find an ending, that I'll know it when I see it.

I suspect, though, that it's the middle that's the tricky part—how to keep going. It's the middle, the long middle, the most of it, that's hardest. That's where we get stuck.

I like marking beginnings and endings, participating in the rituals that identify major life passages. I not only make a big deal of my son's birthdays, but also his half-birthdays: We blow out half-his-age's candles on half a cake and make a half-line on the wall to measure his height.

Maybe these are all endings. A year, a half-year over. Maybe I'm really not so good at beginnings. Although I thought I wanted a traditional wedding—for the ritual of it, the celebration—I never did have one. My partner and I never got married. We say it's because we couldn't find the time in our busy life together to . . . what? To mark the beginning of it? We were too busy living it, right in the middle of it, to decide where it should begin? We don't celebrate anniversaries because we don't have any. So here we are almost two decades later, our relationship not needing to end because it never really began. It just kind of creaks along pleasantly. We grew into each other, became facts of each other's lives. Middle lives, now that we're middle-aged. The long middle.

When I left the hospital, I wore a flower in my hair. It was prettier than a tube up the nose, which is what I had on a few days before. The flower was an emblem of renewal, of the life I was to reenter. I left with a long vertical incision on my stomach, and no colon. From now on my small intestine would do all the work.

The nurse who had yelled at me a few nights ago was being especially friendly. "You're a new woman!" she exclaimed, over-brightly. Maybe she was feeling guilty for chastising me when I got worried that my stomach juices were going the wrong way down the nasal tube. But she was right this time: I was a new woman, with newly configured insides. And I was transformed as much by the experience of it all as I was physically.

Why don't people talk about this? We hear a lot about post-traumatic stress resulting from various causes: the psychological devastation of wars or destructive, abusive relationships. And we hear about people dealing with life-threatening illnesses, about the necessity of counselling and support groups for, say, cancer survivors. But I've never heard anyone characterize an experience as a patient in a Canadian hospital as traumatic in and of itself, as something that one needs to recover from.

And I don't know if I have, quite, recovered. I don't know if I ever really left the place alive.

We put ourselves into the hands of medical people so easily. We have to of course. We trust them with our bodies, our very aliveness, and some of us are taught not to even ask questions. They're the experts after all. I don't mean this facetiously. I know how difficult it is to communicate with people who are outside your area of expertise, your community of discourse. So I don't mean to denigrate doctors. I have an excellent family doctor, and I know many who are wonderful, who treat their patients respectfully and carefully, as if they are knowledgeable about their own bodies and want to stay "in control" of them. Some of my best friends are doctors.

The scar on my stomach isn't just a vertical straight line—it begins above my belly button, veers off to the side of it, and continues the line beneath it. It makes quite a beautiful sweepy point around my navel. If you look at it from the side, it looks like how people draw birds from a distance, like elongated shallow "M"s. When my mother first saw my incision, from beside my hospital bed, she said, "It looks like a bird." She was the one to say it. She made it. Made a bird out of the incision on my tummy, out of the flight path the surgeon's scalpel took. Now I have a special relationship with birds. They're drawn to me. They swoop past me, closer than I've ever known before.

I arrived at the hospital under emergency conditions, when a diverticulum (a pocket in the wall of my colon) burst, and stuff was leaking into my abdominal cavity. The pocket wasn't supposed to be there. I was told a few years before that I would likely have to schedule surgery to remove a portion of my colon, after an X-ray revealed that the lower left portion of it was covered with lots and lots of these little pockets. Either that, or wait for an emergency—then watch out! You could die from a pocket busting open, leaking shit everywhere, just like you could from a burst appendix. I'd been warned.

That I was too young for this kind of condition and it was unusually severe indicated that it was congenital: I'd been born with unusually thick colon walls that just give out and form little pocket-pouches with normal movement. I had suffered many painful bouts of diverticulitis for several years, which is what happens when the little pockets become inflamed or infected. In my case, the state of my colon had no relationship to diet or exercise; there was nothing I could do to keep it in check, even though I tried like hell.

The hole in my pocket turned into a two-week stay on IV antibiotics, exploratory surgery, many tests, and three surgeons. Surgeon One insisted that only the lower-left portion of my bowel was affected, and the reason my pain was on the right side was because it had flopped over. He would perform a very difficult operation—that he was the sole leading expert in, having devised the procedure himself to minimize surgical trauma to the patient's body: go in through my belly button, chop off the offending bit, pull it through, and I would be recovered in no time at all. I should feel lucky to have him on my case. No other surgeon knew as much about bowel surgery, nor were as skilled and brilliant as he, he told me. "I am in control here," he announced, quoting Alexander Haig. And he would fearlessly conquer my colon—and leave me still sick and diseased.

Surgeon Two just didn't know what to do with me. She thought she disagreed with Surgeon One—the tests seemed to suggest that more than just the lower bowel was diseased—but, well, she just didn't know for sure. The nurses said she was under a lot of stress. When I asked her hesitantly, trying to be helpful, "Um, can you take out the different chunks that are diseased? Like, if you had to, how much could you remove?" she gave me a long horrified stare and gasped, "That would be *major* surgery." I was going to have to live with a colon that could rupture at any time and put my life at risk. Oh well.

Surgeon Three was the one who finally saw what was really going on and what could be done about it. Before he sat down in my hospital room and laid out various surgical options to me, I thought I was doomed. No one could do anything for me; this was it. It turned out my *entire* large colon was now diseased! The whole twisting convoluted tube. All five feet of it. From its beginning on the lower left side of my abdomen, through its long tortuous middle, right to its ending, where inside meets outside, the exit point.

Surgeon Three told me I had four options. Option Four was "Don't do anything at all." Although it seemed clear to me which option I should take, he didn't lead me to it. He let me decide. So I was important after all, in all this body stuff. I was so relieved to hear that there were indeed options, that I was going to get through this, I would have hugged him if I could have moved.

My colon-removal surgery was scheduled, and I only had a month or so to get through without more ruptures before I could be rid of the problem once and for all. Apparently there are a few people walking around out there without colons. Who knew? I certainly didn't.

If I did die, and these last three years have been like a dream whose purpose is to ease me gently into the knowledge of my leaving this world, then something just occurred to me: Perhaps this very writing is the final stage. That would make sense. I'm to write my way through this and thus find my way to its conclusion. These words are the passage to a new way of being. If this is the case, I'm writing myself to death. Here is where the transformation is really occurring. It's possible.

I like possibilities. I'm happiest when I have lots of them, of different kinds. I love walking down Commercial Drive, a lively street full of shops, restaurants, cafés—the hub of activity in my urban Vancouver neighbourhood. Just to be out in the world of possibility is fun, not knowing whom I'll run into, what opportunities may come my way, what avenues of creativity and connection will present themselves.

I think I keep things open like this—on the brink of actualizing, liminal—just so I can be more aware of how I can create my world, watch how I'm doing it. If I can recognize that I'm standing on a threshold, then I can step through it consciously, purposefully. When I was told I needed my entire colon removed, I prepared for it as one would who's entering a brand new stage of life. I was literally going to be transformed, reconfigured on the inside. My friends joked that I was losing my guts; I would be the gutless wonder; I'd have a "semi-colon."

But I needed to discover what my colon meant to me and why it had become diseased, unusable. Like everything physical, my body is a metaphor. My colon was for the storage and elimination of waste material, and it didn't work anymore. Maybe I was having trouble knowing how to get rid of things in my life—how to dispose of what's old and worn-out, what's done its time, served its purpose. It's true—although I'm extremely organized, I don't like to throw things away: I have a neat but tightly packed storage area in the basement. Maybe I had to learn how and when to throw stuff out. Make endings. Unambiguous solid endings. Even though I'm not sure I believe in them.

I never thought I believed in victim-hood either. Still don't. But there is an experience for which no other word seems to fit. If being a victim means being helpless while at the mercy of someone or something that has power over you and uses it to mistreat you, then all hospital patients are potential victims, especially the bedridden ones.

I sometimes wonder if my male friends have experienced so many instances of vulnerability and helplessness that I have in my life. I've witnessed violence toward men—seen friends get beaten up, and watched, horrified, unable to do anything. But men just seem to get through the emotional repercussions more easily. Or maybe it just looks that way because of how they're socialized: to at least *seem* unaffected, to not give their emotions much credence, to not feel—or in any case, show—fear. Do women feel victim-hood more acutely than men? Is it part of our very make-up, our bodies, as much as it's created and maintained through culture and language?

Years ago, when an exuberant and happily drunk boyfriend went into the kitchen of the all-night restaurant to ask for some water, our waiter flipped out, dragged him outside and proceeded to strangle him on the sidewalk. When I pleaded desperately with the crazed waiter to let him go, he muttered through clenched teeth, "He is not supposed to go into the kitchen!" I was afraid to do more than tentatively try to push the man off, in case I made him more angry and dangerous. A little crowd formed to watch, until the cops finally came and tore the waiter away, before he squeezed the life out of my boyfriend. But the boyfriend just got up and brushed himself off, and the next day I was more shaken than he was.

When at seventeen I got sick with some undiagnosed abdominal illness and ended up in the hospital, the gynecologist told me I had started on the Pill too young (sixteen was too young), and that was the main problem. It was my fault. My fault for being sexual. He also looked at the books I had on my bedside table: *The Nature of*

Personal Reality (a metaphysical "Seth" book) and a very soft porn comic book, light and amusing, that my sister gave me as a distraction I guess. Dr. Gyno riffled through this bedside litera-ture, and I could see his eyes light up with an aha-I-knew-it! look. "What kind of books are these for a girl?" he thundered.

If I wanted to be healthy of body and mind, I'd better change my reading material too.

Obviously, what was wrong with me had to do with 1) my female body and its wicked sexual yearnings; and, 2) the very strange ideas I invited into my head. That it turned out that a burst ovarian cyst was likely causing the illness didn't matter. I was bad—corrupt—so I was sick. In my heightened emotional state I felt so overwhelmed by the unfairness of his appraisal of me, I broke down crying—which, of course, only confirmed his theory that I needed some kind of psychological help: I was a difficult and confused girl.

I stopped taking the Pill immediately and, for good measure, quit using tampons.

It's true that most of my victim-like experiences are tied into my femininity. I can tell my share of date-rape and sexual assault stories, some terrifying, others upsetting but seemingly par-for-the-course. And when I had my son by emergency C-section, and he was crying in his hospital crib just out of my reach, and I had no way of getting to him—bedridden as I was—I started to cry uncontrollably, helplessly. Again, my female body, slashed as it was above my groin to enable the birth of my baby, was making me vulnerable. The nurses who heeded my distress call exchanged looks that said *Whoa, this one can't handle it; there's something wrong here.* Never mind I'd just been through major surgery as well as childbirth, and my hormones were flooding over. I was being too emotional, irrational.

When my colon crisis brought me to the hospital, Surgeon One was frighteningly reminiscent of Dr. Gyno. He made it seem like it was my fault that I had been given an abdominal CAT scan when I arrived in the ER, and he railed on to his flock of residents from the foot of my gurney, gesticulating dramatically: "She's just cost the taxpayers a couple of grand! And for what? For nothing. A bunch of shadows. They show nothing!" (I was reminded of that guy in *Hogan's Heroes*: "I see nutt-*ink* . . . I hear nutt-*ink*!") He ended up taking himself off my case for two reasons, he told my family doctor: 1) the patient obviously didn't like or trust him because she had cried in his presence for no apparent reason; and 2) he was suspicious of the patient's relationship with a man who was not her husband whom he witnessed holding her hand. In other words: He didn't understand me. I was a difficult and confused woman.

But what does being a victim mean if we somehow create that experience ourselves—if no one really has power over us unless we, ultimately, allow it? It becomes something else: a being vulnerable, putting yourself at the mercy of others. A scary thing to do, and one that has everything to do with trust. But isn't this really how we live our lives? We have to. It has to do with being human. I trust that you understand me. I trust you won't hurt me. I trust that my body won't break down. I trust when I walk down a sidewalk on a busy street that a car won't veer out of control and run me over. I trust that when I can't help myself, you'll help me. I trust that I'll take another breath.

I trust that I'll get through this and out the other side.

The other side: When the Hindu veil of *maya* falls away or when Plato's cave gets all lit up, what do we see? Who's there at the end of the tunnel or at those Christian pearly gates? Where does that overwhelming sense of peace come from that we hear about?

Surely not from leaving our families, friends, lovers. How can I leave my son? How can my mother lose her daughter? *How can the dead and dying really be at peace, knowing that terrible heartbreaking grief is sure to find those they left behind?* How is *that* possible? I've never heard that question asked. And, to me, it's the most pressing one.

Maybe it's because no one *is* left behind. This is what I finally understood on my hospital bed, before Surgeon Three saved me, and after several torturous days and nights contemplating my upcoming death. No one is left behind. The loved ones who greet you at the end of the tunnel, warmly welcoming you to the afterlife, are not just those who died before you. Nope. Everyone is there. It's like what Dorothy finds after she wakes up and sees her neighbours and Auntie Em crowded around her bed, smiling at her: You were there. And you. And you!

All the people whose lives are entangled with ours here are there too, just in a different kind of way. We're there as well, as much as we're here.

There are no endings. Dream on.

If I did die on the operating table, my fading scar is more than an emblem of transformation. It is the secret opening to another world. When I trace its path with my finger, I'm exploring the way to somewhere else. But it doesn't give anything up. As "time" passes, it blends into the colouring of my stomach. Eventually the pathway will become almost hidden, unnoticeable, as its settles into my flesh, in this body.

As I move further away from my experience at the hospital, my life seems to grow more humdrum, less sharply focussed, the edges of objects in the world softening with the scar tissue on my belly.

But I know it's always when you're least aware of something that it hits.

It's only been in this last, third year that I can feel myself getting just a bit *too* comfortable. I am thankful I can still feel the daily discomfort in my new guts, happy to hear my insides rumble like thunder after I eat. (If people nearby hear—and they often do—I just smile, unapologetically.) I am reminded that all is not quite as it seems.

Just under the skin there's something else, as strange as it is familiar.

Any day now.

CONTRIBUTOR NOTES

LUANNE ARMSTRONG is the author of over twelve books, including poetry, novels, and children's books. She is deeply interested in writing about place and nature. Her 2007 book, *Blue Valleys: An Ecological Memoir*, is about growing up in the Kootenays. Luanne lives on her organic heritage farm in the Kootenay region of BC.

DENNIS E. BOLEN, BA (UVic), MFA (UBC), taught in the UBC Creative Writing Program from 1995 to 1997. An arts journalist and critic for nearly thirty years, Dennis' reputation is mainly as a novelist; he is author of five books of fiction, the most recent being *Toy Gun*, which appeared in 2005.

BONNIE BOWMAN's first novel, *Skin*, was the winner of the 22nd annual 3-Day Novel contest and the ReLit award. Her short fiction has appeared in *subTerrain* and *Vancouver Review*, and she has ghostwritten two nonfiction books. She lives in Toronto where she is completing a novel about the Vancouver blues scene and freelancing for lit/trade magazines.

GRANT BUDAY's novels include *A Sack of Teeth*, *White Lung*, and *Rootbound*. He has a new novel, *Dragonflies*, about Odysseus, and a collection of travel stories, *The Curve of the Earth*, the title story of which has been selected for *The Journey Prize Stories 19*. He lives on Mayne Island, B.C.

J. CATES is an ex-Vancouver writer living on Vancouver Island, winner of two MacMillan Bloedel Journalism Awards, whose work has appeared in the *North American Review*, *West Coast Review*, and other periodicals, the *Vancouver Sun* and other newspapers, and who now gets a seniors' discount at Zellers and other stores.

KIM CLARK most often writes from the heart of B.C.'s Sunshine Coast. Disease and desire, mothering and the mundane propel her ongoing journey between poetry and prose. Kim's work can be found in *The Malahat*

Review, Portal, Ascent Aspirations, Wheelhouse, as well as numerous e-zines and other publications in Canada and the U.S.

DOREEN COLMER lives in Maple Ridge, B.C., with her husband and their two sons. Staying healthy keeps Doreen very busy, but in her spare time she relaxes in her garden and craft room. Doreen is working on a book called *where can I find a miracle?* and hopes her story will inspire others.

BEVERLEY A. FEATHER's 120-acre farm on Vancouver Island is the background for her humorous stories published in *Country* and *Country Woman* magazines. With her sister, Beverley has co-written two amateur detective novels, and she is presently putting her stories together for a book from the farmwoman's point of view. She works as a teacher in Nanaimo.

ALAN GIRLING lives in Richmond, B.C. His writing has appeared in such literary periodicals as *Lichen, Hobart, The MacGuffin, Smokelong Quarterly,* and *River Walk Journal,* and on CBC radio. He recently won Vancouver Co-op Radio's Community Dreams Poetry Contest, and his play, *Whatever Happened to Tom Dudkowski* was produced for Vancouver's 2007 Walking Fish Festival.

DENISE HALPERN lives in Vancouver after spending many years Down Under where she was involved in theatre. Her poetry and nonfiction have appeared in Australian periodicals, and she has a play in the collection *Life Stages.* "Seeing it Through" is a monologue that was first performed at the Vancouver Fringe Festival.

JANIS HARPER is a college and university English instructor, a Vancouver actor, and singer-songwriter. She has co-founded two local periodicals and published journalism and scholarship. Her poetry and prose have appeared in Canadian literary journals, including *Room of One's Own, Contemporary Verse 2,* and *Tessera,* and in the international fiction anthology, *Lost on Purpose: Women in the City.*

MELODY HESSING lives in Vancouver, teaches sociology in post-secondary institutions (most recently Douglas College and UBC), and has written numerous scholarly articles and books. Nowadays, creative writing projects—nonfiction, short stories, and skeins of poetry—entice her, sometimes as much as mountains. She strongly suspects that the mind-body dichotomy is a fiction.

CRYSTAL HURDLE teaches creative writing and English at Capilano College in North Vancouver. Her book, *After Ted & Sylvia: Poems*, is about Plath and Hughes; and her poetry has been published widely in Canadian journals, including *Canadian Literature*, *Fireweed*, and *The Dalhousie Review*. The letters in this anthology are from a manuscript in progress, *Cat Scratch Fever*.

EMMA KIVISILD is a writer, performer, and artist living in Vancouver, proud to have been part of two KickstART! festivals. As Lizard Jones, she is a member of the award-winning collective Kiss & Tell. Her novel *Two Ends of Sleep*, about living with MS, was published in 1997.

ADRIENNE MERCER lives in Nanaimo, B.C. She writes creative nonfiction, fiction, and poetry, and is a member of the Big Picture Window writers' group. Adrienne is also the author of *Rebound*, a young adult novel set in the West Kootenay village of Nakusp.

RUTH MURDOCH, an artist, writer, and registered art therapist, lives rurally near Smithers, B.C. Her paintings, sculptures, and fibre arts have been shown at the Smithers Art Gallery, and her poems are published in *Creekstones: Words and Images*. She believes passionately in the power of image and metaphor.

SUSAN OLDING's essays have been short-listed for two Western Magazine Awards and a National Magazine Award, and she has won both the *Event* and *Prairie Fire* Creative Nonfiction contests. She lives with her family in Kingston, Ontario, where she teaches at the Queen's University Writing Centre and with the Department of Film and Media.

STEPHEN OSBORNE is the editor and co-founder of *Geist* magazine. He has received several writing awards, including the CBC nonfiction prize and the first Vancouver Arts Writing and Publishing Award. Some of his personal essays have been collected in *Ice & Fire: Dispatches from the New World*.

JANE SILCOTT's writing has been published in *The Malahat Review, Prairie Fire, Room of One's Own, Contemporary Verse 2, Geist,* and *Utne*. In 2005, she won second place in the CBC Literary Awards for nonfiction. Jane lives with her family in Vancouver, where she teaches and writes and looks at mountains from her attic writing office.

BOB WAKULICH's work has appeared in journals, periodicals, and anthologies in North America and Europe, as well as on CBC Radio and in cyberspace. He currently lives in Cranbrook, B.C., with his wife and three cats, teaches at the local college, and writes a humour column for the *Cranbrook Daily Townsman*.

BRAD ZEMBIC is a Vancouver-based travel writer and book reviewer. His work appears in both national and international newspapers, including the *Georgia Straight, Vancouver Sun, Edmonton Journal,* and *Cape Argus* in Cape Town, South Africa. When not wandering the African veld, Brad teaches in a high school program for the deaf in the Fraser Valley.

THIS BOOK WAS PRINTED ON 100% POST-CONSUMER, OLD-GROWTH FRIENDLY PAPER.